in_focus

Health

AN ECOSYSTEM APPROACH

in_focus

IDRC's *In_Focus* Collection tackles current and pressing issues in sustainable international development. Each publication distills IDRC's research experience with an eye to drawing out important lessons, observations, and recommendations for decision-makers and policy analysts. Each also serves as a focal point for an IDRC Web site that probes more deeply into the issue, and is constructed to serve the differing information needs of IDRC's various readers. A full list of *In_Focus* Web sites may be found at **www.idrc.ca/in_focus**. Each *In_Focus* book may be browsed and ordered online at **www.idrc.ca/booktique**.

IDRC welcomes any feedback on this publication.

Please direct your comments to The Publisher at **pub@idrc.ca**.

Health

AN ECOSYSTEM APPROACH

by **Jean Lebel**

INTERNATIONAL DEVELOPMENT RESEARCH CENTRE
Ottawa • Cairo • Dakar • Montevideo • Nairobi • New Delhi • Singapore

Published by the International Development Research Centre
PO Box 8500, Ottawa, ON, Canada K1G 3H9
http://www.idrc.ca

© International Development Research Centre 2003

National Library of Canada Cataloguing in Publication

Lebel, Jean, 1963-
    Health : an ecosystem approach / Jean Lebel.

Issued also in French under title: La santé, une approche écosystémique.

ISBN 1-55250-012-8

1. Environmental health.
2. Environmental health — Research.
3. Public health.
I. International Development Research Centre (Canada)
II. Title.

RA565.L42 2003   363.7   C2003-902434-2

IDRC Books endeavours to produce environmentally friendly publications.
All paper used is recycled as well as recyclable. All inks and coatings are
vegetable-based products.

**This publication may be read online at www.idrc.ca/booktique,
and serves as the focal point for an IDRC thematic Web site on
ecosystem approaches to human health: www.idrc.ca/ecohealth.**

Contents

Foreword — Pierre Dansereau ➤ **vii**

Preface ➤ **xi**

Chapter 1. The Issue ➤ **1**

Can people remain healthy in a world that is sick? Many ecological disasters can be directly traced to careless exploitation of the environment, with human beings becoming both perpetrator and victim. Our health closely mirrors the health of our surroundings. This is the basis of the Ecohealth approach, which recognizes the inextricable links between humans and their biophysical, social, and economic environments, and that these links are reflected in a population's state of health.

From Stockholm to Johannesburg . 3
Ecosystem health = human health . 5
Beyond the biophysical . 6

Chapter 2. The Approaches ➤ **9**

Reconciling an ecosystem's health with the health of its human inhabitants is a new area of research, requiring input from scientists, community groups, decision-makers, and other interested parties. This chapter describes the three methodological pillars of the Ecohealth approach: transdisciplinarity, community participation, and gender equity.

A transdisciplinary framework . 10
Defining a common language . 13
The challenges of transdisciplinarity . 16
A participatory approach . 18
Increasing participation . 21
Challenges of the participatory approach . 22
Gender and equity . 25

Chapter 3. Lessons and Successes ➤ 31

Agriculture, mining, and urban growth: three areas with powerful impacts on both human health and the environment, particularly in the developing countries of the South. Research employing the Ecohealth approach has yielded promising results in each of these areas.

Mining . 32
Agriculture . 41
The urban environment . 43
Comprehensible results, sustainable solutions . 50

Chapter 4. Recommendations and Future Directions ➤ 57

The Ecohealth approach presents new challenges and opportunities for researchers, community groups, and decision-makers. Decision-makers, in particular, can benefit by drawing from the results of Ecohealth research to formulate policies and solutions that are both immediately visible and sustainable over the long term.

Early recognition . 57
Challenging scientists . 60
Challenges for decision-makers . 60
The promise of the Ecohealth approach . 61

Appendix: Sources and Resources ➤ 67

The Publisher ➤ 85

Foreword

Ecohealth at last!

For an ecologist of early vintage, the emergence of ecohealth is an historical step. It involves the appropriation of ecological knowledge and methodology by the prescriptive sector of the social sciences. Indeed, until the fifties, ecology was monopolized by biology: the International Biological Programme (IBP) had clearly confined its scope by exclusively aiming at the behaviour of plants and animals "in the wild." This position was justified by the fact that very few explicitly ecological research papers were set within man-occupied spaces.

Forest ecology had nevertheless taken its stance, even if it was geared to economic considerations. Agricultural ecology had made very few inroads. Human ecology, in spite of the excellence of its founder's treaty (Thomas Park in 1924), remained in the shadows. Urban ecology hardly existed.

One had to wait for the dramatic entry of anthropologists, sociologists, economists, architects, and urbanists to break the monopoly of Biology. This master science, not unlike Physics, was submerged in "the heart of matter," in molecular biology. Botanists and zoologists no longer breathed the maritime air, nor wet their feet, nor submitted to tropical heat or alpine cold. They seemed to think that the tasks of taxonomy and field ecology were done.

The human sciences, on the other hand, were justly appropriating the arsenal of facts and processes discovered by the ecologists and the interpretations that they had offered. On the occasion of a symposium (*Future Environments of North America*) held by the Conservation Foundation of Washington in 1965, the great economist Kenneth Boulding had vehemently exclaimed: "You ecologists, you don't know what a good thing you have!"

Health is not the absence of illness in Jean Lebel's perspective. It is better defined as a harmonious participation in the resources of the environment, which allows individuals the full play of their functions and aptitudes. It can hardly maintain itself if the exploitants that we are do not assume full responsibility for a vigilant economy.

This generation is in the act of gravely menacing the heritage of its descendents. The present text ably describes the damages that are visible at the planetary level. It emphasizes the help that IDRC offers, at the four corners of the planet, in spaces where uncontrolled natality inhibits a traditional wisdom that must adjust to the perception of science.

This is a big step beyond missionary paternalism. However, one might have welcomed a parallel environmental problematic of the industrial countries with that of the Third World to whom an avoidance of our errors should be assured.

A reading of this book is so very profitable that one wishes to go beyond its premises. If the author should be more in the foreground, he would hardly be blamed. Should he also retrace his own itinerary, he would all the better engage in a perspective of Canadian accomplishments.

In an epoch where the aid of industrialized countries to areas of poverty aims at an increase therein of their purchasing power, and not a reinvestment of profits achieved, it is very useful to read such an objective account as this one. Jean Lebel, actor and witness, offers us a truly innovative analysis.

Pierre Dansereau
Professor of Ecology
Institut des sciences de l'environnement
Université du Québec à Montréal

Pierre Dansereau, professor emeritus of ecology at the Université du Québec à Montréal, has had a long career, from the forties onward, in teaching and in research. He has occupied various positions at the universities of Montréal, Michigan, Columbia (New York), Lisbon, and Dunedin (New Zealand). He was assistant director of the New York Botanical Garden and is the author of several books and other publications in the fields of plant taxonomy and genetics, plant ecology, biogeography, and human ecology.

THE ISSUE

Preface

Human health cannot be considered in isolation. It depends highly on the quality of the environment in which people live: for people to be healthy, they need healthy environments.

The Ecosystem Approaches to Human Health program of Canada's International Development Research Centre (IDRC) — the result of many years of collaboration between Canada and the countries in the South — is an innovative response to human health problems resulting from the transformation or high-risk management of either the environment or human health. This program is based on what has become known as the Ecohealth approach.

The purpose of this book is to introduce the Ecohealth approach, provide examples of how it is applied, and draw a few lessons that should encourage its use by decision-makers. This approach to human health places human beings at the centre: the aim is to achieve lasting improvements in human health by maintaining or improving the environment. Its proponents work for both people and the environment.

At IDRC, the Ecosystem Approaches to Human Health program reflects many years of evolution in support for health research. In the early days, the research supported was largely biomedical: vaccines, disease-control strategies, and contraception. Later, IDRC began to take the environment and the community into account. In 1990, the program was called Health, Society, and Environment but, although it involved specialists from different disciplines working together, it sought only to improve human health, not the environment.

IDRC created the Ecohealth program in 1996. This innovative program proposed inviting scientists, decision-makers, and community members to work toward improving the community's health by improving the environment. This was the first step in adopting a deliberately transdisciplinary approach in an IDRC program. Since then, the program has supported some 70 projects in about 30 countries in Latin America, Africa, the Middle East, and Asia.

The Ecohealth approach is anthropocentric — managing the ecosystem revolves around seeking the optimal balance for human health and well-being, rather than simply on environmental protection. Thus, its objective is not to preserve the environment as it was before human settlements appeared. The presence of human beings creates a new dynamic whereby people's social and economic aspirations need to be considered, particularly since people have the power to control, develop, and use their environment in a sustainable way, or to abuse it. That is an original aspect of this approach.

Another original aspect is the adoption of a research process that is not restricted to scientists, so that the knowledge acquired can be integrated into people's lives. The effectiveness and sustainability of these actions are at the heart of our concerns. The challenge is meeting human needs without modifying or jeopardizing the ecosystem in the long term — and, ideally, even improving it.

The many inquiries we have received have convinced us of the importance of presenting our ecosystem approaches to human health. That is the main purpose of this book. Also, by sharing research findings and lessons, IDRC hopes to contribute to the development of a vision and tools that decision-makers can use, in collaboration with communities, to formulate health and environmental policies.

I would like to warmly thank all the members of the Ecosystem Approaches to Human Health team at IDRC, particularly Roberto Bazzani, Ana Boischio, Renaud De Plaen, Kathleen Flynn-Dapaah, Jean-Michel Labatut, Zsofia Orosz, and Andrés Sanchez, for their contribution to this book, as well as Gilles Forget and Don Peden for their work during the first years of our program. I am also deeply grateful to all of the Ecohealth project participants throughout the world who have helped to develop ecosystem approaches to human health and are working energetically to put them into practice. This book would not have been possible without their collaboration. Finally, I am grateful to Danielle Ouellet, editor of *Découvrir* magazine in Montréal, who produced the first draft of the book, and to Jean-Marc Fleury and his team in IDRC's Communications Division for their patience in seeing this project through to completion.

Jean Lebel

Jean Lebel earned a master's degree in occupational health sciences and a graduate diploma in occupational hygiene from McGill University in Montréal, as well as a PhD in environmental sciences (1996) from the Université du Québec à Montréal (UQAM). He is currently team leader of IDRC's Ecosystem Approaches to Human Health program initiative. As an environmental health specialist, he spent of much of the four years of study leading to his PhD in the Amazon region of Brazil. With a transdisciplinary research team, he studied the effects of low-level contamination, especially by mercury, on human health. In April 2001, he received the first UQAM Prix Reconnaissance from its Faculty of Sciences for the work he "has pioneered by helping developing countries preserve the balance of their ecosystems and protect the health of their citizens."

Chapter 1

The Issue

Can people remain healthy in a world that is sick? What sort of environment are we going to leave behind for our children? How can we exploit nonrenewable resources without harming our health? What are the realistic compromises needed between the short-term benefits of exploiting natural resources and the long-term costs to the environment and human health? How can we live in overcrowded cities without poisoning each other?

In the mountainous regions of the Andes, the Himalayas, or Ethiopia, impoverished peasants eke out their living from the land and occasionally have enough left over to sell at the market. Their farming techniques often lead to soil degradation. Sometimes they result in collective poisoning because of the misuse of pesticides. In the Amazon, families struggling to clear their little plot of land in the forest release mercury that has been locked up in the soil for hundreds of thousands of years. Through a long process, this mercury becomes toxic and finds its way into their bodies and that of their children. People in Mexico City and Kathmandu, despite their poverty or perhaps because of it, can produce enough pollution to reduce their life expectancy. In the mineral-rich regions of the Andes or India, the local mining industry provides much-needed jobs, but sometimes at the cost of poisoning the soil, which contaminates the miners' food and that of their families.

In developing countries, the longstanding environmentally harmful effects of deforestation and overgrazing are now being aggravated by the disastrous consequences of industrialization and modernization. The ecosystems suffer the combined assault. At the beginning, exploiting an ecosystem automatically reduces its resilience or ability to rebound. When that ecosystem also has to sustain a rapidly growing human population reduced to adopting basic survival strategies, the ecosystem's resilience can be lethally undermined. But even before that, a series of perverse mechanisms can be set in motion, endangering the health of populations.

The issue that ecosystem approaches to human health — the Ecohealth approach — address is no less than humanity's place in its environment. As Mariano Bonet, the leader of a rehabilitation project in the oldest section of Havana, puts it: "The Ecohealth approach recognizes that there are inextricable links between humans and their biophysical, social, and economic environments that are reflected in an individual's health."

The ecosystem approach to human health is tied to the overall development of ecology during the second half of the 20th century. The emergence of this discipline has influenced the thinking of physicians like Dr Bonet, but also of many other specialists, including environmentalists, urban planners, agronomists, biologists, and sociologists, both in developing countries and the industrialized world. In the beginning, ecology adopted a perspective that was largely based on the biophysical aspects of an ecosystem. In fact, some people still consider ecology as a means of restoring ecosystems to their primitive state. Faced with the reality of a global population of some 6.3 billion people that is well on its way to 9 or 10 billion within 50 years, however, it is difficult to exclude people from the ecological equation. An increasing number therefore now include human communities in the description of contemporary ecosystems.

For those with a holistic vision, humanity with its aspirations and its cultural, social, and economic universe is at the heart of the ecosystem, on an equal footing with biophysical parameters. The living and the nonliving elements of nature interact toward a dynamic equilibrium that, better managed, should ensure the sustainable development of human communities.

From Stockholm to Johannesburg

In 1972, for the first time, the environment appeared on the world's agenda at the United Nations Conference on the Environment in Stockholm. From there was born the notion of "eco-development." Then, in 1987, the Brundtland report — *Our Common Future* — introduced the idea of sustainable development as "development that meets the needs of the present without compromising the ability of future generations to meet their own needs." Although this acknowledged the role of people in environmental change, it took another five years before the connection between the environment and human health was clearly made at a major international conference.

The United Nations Conference on the Environment and Development in Rio de Janeiro in 1992 advanced the concept of sustainable development and specified the place of men and women in such development: "Human beings are at the centre of concerns for sustainable development."

Agenda 21, which the governments of 185 countries adopted at this conference in Brazil, clearly spelled out the close link between human health and the environment. In fact, an entire chapter of Agenda 21 is devoted to the protection and promotion of human health. Simply put, if people are not in good health, development cannot be sustainable. Agenda 21 highlighted the connection between poverty and underdevelopment on the one hand, and the connection between environmental protection and natural resource management on the other. This new notion captured international attention. Agenda 21 also identified the many partners involved in implementing these measures: children, women, youth, indigenous peoples, workers, farmers, scientists, teachers, business people, decision-makers, and nongovernmental organizations (NGOs).

The World Summit on Sustainable Development in Johannesburg, in August–September 2002, placed much more emphasis on the social and economic aspects of sustainable development. Health was one of its five priorities. The World Health Organization (WHO) has taken responsibility for an action plan on health and the environment. This plan deals with several issues at the intersection of health, the environment, and development, such as water contamination, air pollution, and the management of toxic substances.

IDRC's Ecosystem Approaches to Human Health program participates in this movement toward heightened concern with the links between health and the environment. This program was created at the crossroads of the development of practices in public health and in ecosystem health. The program takes a holistic, dynamic approach that evolves with the experience of its partners in both South and North who are working on development issues affecting local communities.

Ecosystem health = human health

Discoveries in health and progress in healing techniques have considerably reduced the incidence of infectious disease in industrialized countries and, to a lesser extent, in developing countries. The biomedical approach to health is based on methods of diagnosing and treating specific pathologies: one pathogen = one disease. This approach, however, does not take into account the connections between disease and socioeconomic factors such as poverty and malnutrition, and even less of the connections between disease and the environment in which sick people live. In general, the biomedical approach to human health displays the same lack of attention to the impact of cultural factors on high-risk behaviour and the particular vulnerability of certain groups.

Despite some progress, environmental factors still dramatically affect the health of many people. WHO estimates that approximately three million children die each year from environment-related causes and more than one million adults die of work-related illnesses or injuries. Between 80 and 90 percent of diarrhea cases are caused by environmental factors. In developing countries, between 2.0 and 3.5 billion people use fuels that give off smoke and other harmful substances. In rural areas, poor animal husbandry practices result in the spread of animal-transmitted diseases and resistance to antibiotics.

In many ways, traditional methods have failed to improve the well-being, health, and sanitary conditions of people living in the South. These failures concern scientists, governments, international organizations, and donor agencies. Needed are changes in programs and policies and the vision to look beyond conventional health practices. To start, we need to look beyond the biophysical characteristics of ecosystems.

Beyond the biophysical

Predicting the health consequences of the many interactions between different ecosystem components is enormously challenging. Most agree that these interactions are highly complex and, to cover more than just biophysical parameters, researchers will need to review their research methods and be open to new forms of cooperation.

The impact of environmental factors on human health — particularly on the health of people in the South — is now well established. In North Africa, for example, 70 percent of wild plants have a household use, either as medication or food. But despite its importance, African forestland, which covers 22 percent of the continent, lost more than 50 million hectares between 1990 and 2000. For its part, Latin America contributed 190 of the 418 million hectares of forests lost throughout the world during the last 30 years. The loss of biological diversity associated with this kind of disappearance may have direct consequences on human health since about 75 percent of the world's population uses traditional medicines, derived directly from natural sources. In the "new" urban environments, sewerage systems, where they exist, overflow with the household and industrial wastes produced by city populations that are expanding by 2 percent per year.

In this context, it is impossible to improve the environment without including the human population, with its inherent social, cultural, and economic concerns, in the management of resources (Figure 1). In fact, the more we try to stabilize ecosystems by external measures, such as irrigation, drainage, fertilizers or pesticides, the more we diminish their ability to regenerate themselves. A sectoral approach is no longer adequate: co-management of human activity and the environment is essential. This challenge requires that disciplines draw together to study the human–environment relationship.

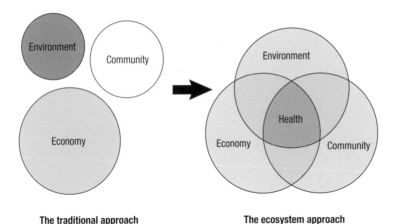

| The traditional approach | The ecosystem approach |

Figure 1. The ecosystem approach gives equal importance to environmental management, economic factors, and community aspirations. Traditional methods focus more on the latter two, to the detriment of the environment (adapted from Hancock 1990).

The economy, the environment, and community needs all affect the health of the ecosystem. Focusing on just one of these factors to the detriment of others compromises ecosystem sustainability. The Ecohealth approach is thus part of the sustainable development process. It promotes positive action on the environment that improves community well-being and health. The underlying hypothesis of the Ecohealth approach is that the programs it generates will be less costly than many medical treatments or primary health care interventions.

Societies and their leaders often face a difficult choice: resort to simple, quick, and sometimes expensive means of tackling complex problems, means that sometimes fail in the longer term — such as the use of DDT as a magic bullet to fight malaria — or invest in socially and economically effective long-term sustainable development. To properly address the sources of environmental degradation and to work with all of the relevant stakeholders, it is essential to go beyond simple health or environmental perspectives.

Chapter 2

The Approaches

Striking a balance between the health of ecosystems and of the people who live in them calls for a new research framework — a framework that includes not only scientists, but also community members, government representatives, and other stakeholders.

The new research framework proposed in this book and described in detail in this chapter is called the "ecosystem approach to human health" — Ecohealth, for short. However, before describing this approach, it must be stressed that each Ecohealth activity or project inherently involves three groups of participants: researchers and other specialists; community members, including ordinary citizens, peasants, fisherfolk, miners, and city-dwellers; and decision-makers. This category includes everyone with decision-making power — not only representatives of government or other key stakeholder groups but also those with informal influence based on their knowledge, experience, and reputation. The goal of each Ecohealth activity is to include this trio.

In addition to requiring the participation of these three groups, the Ecohealth approach is based on three methodological pillars: transdisciplinarity, participation, and equity.

→ **Transdisciplinarity** implies an inclusive vision of ecosystem-related health problems. This requires the full participation of each of the three groups mentioned above and validates their complete inclusion.

→ **Participation** aims to achieve consensus and cooperation, not only within the community, scientific, and decision-making groups but also among them.

→ **Equity** involves analyzing the respective roles of men and women, and of various social groups. The gender dimension recognizes that men and women have different responsibilities and different degrees of influence on decisions: it is therefore important to take gender into account when dealing with access to resources. For their part, various castes, ethnic groups, and social classes often live in completely separate worlds: this isolation has its own repercussions on health and access to resources.

The following sections discuss each of these pillars and present examples of their application.

A transdisciplinary framework

When scientists from various disciplines involve both individuals and decision-makers from the communities they study, we can say that they are operating within a transdisciplinary framework. Scientists using a transdisciplinary approach send a clear signal that they will look at various aspects of a problem by closely involving the local population as well as decision-makers in their work.

When social problems are articulated in questions that can be addressed in a scientific process, communities are able to express what they expect from scientists and decision-makers. This, in turn, leads to "socially robust" solutions. These are just two of the many potential benefits of the transdisciplinary approach.

Transdisciplinarity therefore implies the participation not only of scientists but also of community representatives and other actors who, in addition to possessing particular knowledge of the problem at hand, have a role and a stake in its solution. Such "non-scientists" often belong to an NGO or government agency. The transdisciplinary approach gives them the right to be heard and thereby share their experiences, knowledge, and expectations.

The trandisciplinary approach differs from the unidisciplinary research that characterizes the experimental sciences, such as chemistry and physics, and the theoretical sciences, such as mathematics. It also differs from the interdisciplinary approach, which studies phenomena at the intersection of two disciplines that are usually close to each other, such as the overlap between biology and chemistry that has given rise to biochemistry. Nor is it equivalent to multidisciplinarity, in which researchers from different disciplines work side by side, thereby enriching their own understanding as a result of their colleagues' input, but where coordination does not necessarily lead to integrated actions.

The complexity of the interactions between the various economic, social, and environmental components of an ecosystem requires integrated research strategies that go beyond multidisciplinary frameworks (Figure 2).

A transdisciplinary approach enables researchers from different disciplines and key actors to develop a common vision, while preserving the richness and strength of their respective areas of knowledge. By adopting this approach at the outset the research team avoids carrying out parallel studies whose results are pooled

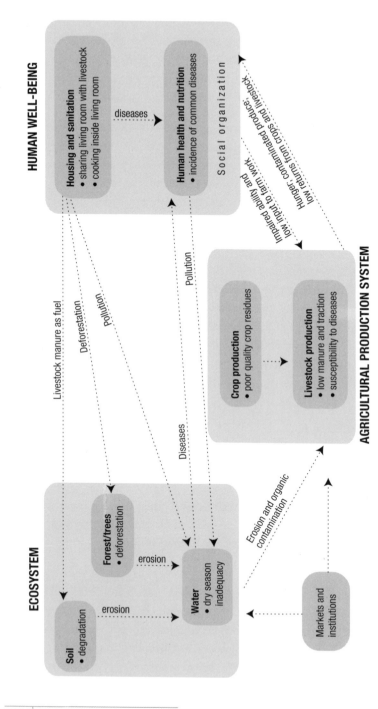

HUMAN WELL-BEING

Housing and sanitation
• sharing living room with livestock
• cooking inside living room

diseases

Human health and nutrition
• incidence of common diseases

Social organization

ECOSYSTEM

Soil
• degradation

Forest/trees
• deforestation

Water
• dry season inadequacy

erosion

erosion

Livestock manure as fuel

Deforestation

Pollution

Diseases

Pollution

AGRICULTURAL PRODUCTION SYSTEM

Crop production
• poor quality crop residues

Livestock production
• low manure and traction
• susceptibility to diseases

Impaired ability to input to farm work; low returns from crops and livestock; Hunger; contaminated produce;

Erosion and organic contamination

Markets and institutions

Figure 2. **Human well-being in Yubdo–Lagabato, Ethiopia, is closely linked to the condition of agroecological system (adapted from ILRI 2001).**

only at the end. The integration of knowledge and the adoption of a common language take place while the problem is being defined — that's the core of the transdisciplinary approach.

Defining a common language

The case of mercury pollution in the Amazon (see Box 9, p. 52) well illustrates transdisciplinarity's contribution. The initial research focused exclusively on the role of mining — specifically, small-scale gold mining in which mercury was used to separate the gold from the ore. However, it was discovered that exposure to methyl mercury, a toxic derivative of mercury, did not diminish in proportion to the distance from the mine. Thanks to the input of a broad range of specialists in the fields of fisheries, aquatic ecology, toxicology, agriculture, human health, social sciences, and nutrition, as well as the participation of the communities concerned, it was finally discovered that local agricultural practices caused the problem.

In this particular case, a transdisciplinary framework was not established at the outset, but was introduced progressively. The research team's experiments in integrating the knowledge of specialists, local populations, and local actors gradually gave rise to a transdisciplinary approach.

The projects supported by IDRC's Ecohealth program have often started with multidisciplinary teams. This has been an important means of achieving transdisciplinarity. These projects have succeeded in broadening the horizons of several researchers used to concentrating on their own discipline while working in parallel with others. Despite this progress, however, widening areas of research does not always result in transdisciplinarity. Several projects began by producing essentially classic outcomes: a diagnosis of degradation of the environment or of human health, for instance, made without proposing concrete measures to improve health. Moreover, participating populations often became simple sources of information rather than full participants in the project.

Since 1997, IDRC has therefore systematically supported the organization of preproject workshops that give scientists, local authorities, and community members the opportunity to pool their knowledge and interests. This blending of information, ideas, and needs makes it possible to define research objectives that clearly reflect the community's real priorities. At the same time, the workshop specifies expectations, because it is just as important to state what the people will not receive. Once the community accepts that a hospital will not be built or that additional grants will be obtained, it becomes easier to reach consensus on what the community will actually get out of the project.

One such workshop, organized in the Mwea region north of Nairobi, Kenya, played a crucial role in a malaria-control project (see Box 6, p. 43). The initial workshop brought together 23 participants from 17 organizations representing government, local communities, rice producers, and various churches.

Several complex issues were involved and no single discipline was adequate to provide the knowledge needed to improve the environmental and health situation. Therefore, the scientific team assembled consisted of eight disciplines: a pathologist, a physician specialized in parasitology, a public health specialist, an agronomist, a veterinarian, an anthropologist, a sociologist, and a statistician. Once the issues were clearly defined, the team members integrated their knowledge and expertise into the research program. As mandated by the transdisciplinary approach, each specialist was required to work with representatives of other disciplines and to integrate the knowledge and concerns of nonscientific partners.

It is noteworthy that the composition of teams dealing with a problem like malaria can vary depending on location. Naturally, mosquitoes will always be a factor, but the local sociocultural and political context will rarely be the same. The composition of the research team will therefore vary according to the region's particular needs. That is why project planning — a process that can take up to one or two years — is so important.

To launch the process, the preproject workshops have proven their worth by bringing together scientists, community members, and political actors. One workshop consists of brainstorming between specialists and representatives of the groups most concerned. Together, they define a vision and common language that subsequently facilitates the conversion of research results into applicable, sustainable action programs. Anyone seeking a quick fix to social and environmental problems abstain: the substantial preliminary planning required for an Ecohealth project will test your patience.

The success of a preproject workshop can be measured by how easily the teams can get started. For example, a team working on the connections between malaria and farming practices in the Fayoum region of Egypt ran into major conceptual difficulties very early on in the project. Fortunately, the preproject workshop gave them the opportunity to integrate into their definition of the problem a wide range of social, anthropological, economic, behavioural, epidemiological, pedagogical, microbiological, hydrological, medical, and policy-related aspects. They were then able to rethink the project, go beyond a strictly agronomic and ecotoxicological framework, and adopt a more holistic view of the situation.

After consulting the local population, a project that initially focused on malaria was expanded to include two other equally important problems: the presence of gastrointestinal parasites and schistosomiasis. (Schistosomiasis, also known as bilharziasis, is a parasitic infection of the intestine, liver, blood vessels, or urinary organs.)

In addition, representatives of the country's health and agricultural ministries became keenly interested because their knowledge was taken into consideration when defining the project. What's more, a local NGO saw this project as an excellent opportunity to link social development — the NGO's mission — with the sustainable development of the local ecosystem. Representatives of this NGO quickly became the project's main driving force in the field.

In less than a year this transdisciplinary team has set in motion a research project involving almost 2 000 people, a fifth of the village population. These people make up a representative sample that is tested every six months for malaria, schistosomiasis, and gastrointestinal parasites. The team combines this information with its analyses of soil moisture content, soil erosion, and salinization. This data is also analyzed in terms of the socioeconomic and political characteristics of the various community groups.

The initial findings show that agricultural practices, which have traditionally been considered to be the cause of these diseases, are not the only factors responsible. For example, a direct link has been discovered between cases of schistosomiasis and gastro-enteritis and the proximity of the many small sun- or oven-dried mud brick manufacturing operations in the region. The children who work in these factories show much higher levels of infection than others.

The scientists involved generally agree that the initial success of projects using an Ecohealth approach is partly due to the experience acquired in preproject workshops.

The challenges of transdisciplinarity

Even though, in theory, transdisciplinarity now enjoys high standing in the scientific community, it still remains a challenge for each Ecohealth project. Going beyond one's own discipline requires a great capability for synthesis as well as sensitivity to the strengths and limitations of others. Suceeding in a transdisciplinary initiative requires defining a research protocol (Box 1), finding ways of integrating the community in problem definition, and ascribing appropriate importance to the various ecosystem components.

Box 1. | A transdisciplinary research protocol

A. The groups or key players

➤ Scientists wanting to work directly for community well-being.

➤ A community ready to collaborate in a development process that uses research as a tool.

➤ Decision-makers who are able to devote time, knowledge, and expertise to a process of consensus-building

B. The steps

➤ Establish dialogue among the key players through informal meetings and exchange of letters and emails.

➤ Solicit the financial support required to fund problem definition in a pre-project workshop that brings together key players.

➤ Organize a preproject workshop to

  – Define the problem based on the views and knowledge of each group (focus group, maps, interaction, data)

  – Identify common areas of concern

  – Agree on common objectives

  – Specify the methodological approach of each group or actor

  – Define roles and responsibilities

  – Establish a schedule for team meetings.

➤ Iterate protocols on the basis of the results achieved.

➤ Translate research results into concrete action programs.

➤ Ensure the project's long-term sustainability and monitor progress.

Equally challenging is assembling a team and organizing the work of members from extremely different disciplines. In agricultural projects, for example, research teams are still mostly made up of medical specialists and agronomists. In general, these teams only have one social scientist, responsible simultaneously for the sociocultural aspects of the research, including gender and equity issues, and for implementing the participatory methodology.

Supervising a transdisciplinary project is all the more difficult when the original concept stems from a particular discipline and the researchers are not aware of the transdisciplinary nature of the problem. It is therefore only to be expected that the development of transdisciplinary projects is time-consuming. Funders of Ecohealth projects need to calculate the financial requirements accordingly. Make no bones about it, Ecohealth projects require large amounts of financial and human resources.

A participatory approach

An extensive body of experience, including that acquired in IDRC projects, has shown that there can be no development without community involvement. This is a main feature of the ecosystem approach to human health. Participatory research gives equal weight to both local and scientific knowledge. Feasible solutions are identified by exchanging knowledge and jointly analyzing problems. Projects must take local knowledge, concerns, and needs into account. This requires involving the local population in the research conducted in their community. This type of research goes beyond the simple verification of hypotheses and leads to action.

The participatory approach targets community representatives and involves them directly in the research process. It takes the different social groups into account and facilitates negotiations.

Box 2. | Ethiopian peasants articulate their problems

Yubdo Legabato, a village of some 5 000 inhabitants 80 km west of Addis Ababa in Ethiopia, was chosen as a test case for the Ecohealth approach because of iits extreme poverty, the poor health of its inhabitants, and the apparent intractability of its many problems.

The researchers sought to determine whether the people of Yubdo Legabato could articulate their health problems and formulate action plans to solve them within a transdisciplinary framework. The villagers were therefore asked what criteria they used to assess their own health, what factors caused their problems, and what actions they thought they could take to improve the situation.

Initially, the problem most frequently mentioned was a shortage of food. The farmers attributed their problems to *dhabuu*, which means "not having enough" in the Oromiya language. However, after the researchers encouraged the peasants to identify broader causes for their problems, they cited several other factors: lack of fodder, lack of water during the dry season, soil erosion, and a resurgence of malaria, measles, and gastroenteritis.

The Ecohealth team then helped the villagers make the connection between their farming practices, the use of natural resources, and their health. The results of this study show that agriculture, the environment, human health, and nutrition are closely interrelated. They highlight the need to adopt a holistic approach to the factors that are detrimental to human well-being. For example, the practice of sleeping on dirt floors with the animals during the cold season, when the average night temperature falls to 5°C, could explain many of the population's infections. But other reasons also underlie this habit, particularly the insecure land-tenure system. Why should people invest in constructing beds when they might be forced to clear out at a moment's notice, leaving everything behind?

The researchers encouraged the farmers to think of constructive changes they could make themselves, instead of waiting for outside help. As soon as the people realized that some of their practices were harmful to their health, they took matters into their own hands. Abiye Astatke, an agricultural engineer with the International Livestock Research Institute (ILRI), points out that since then "People built different houses for their livestock, people built a separate room for cooking their food, and also started building raised platforms for sleeping."

The researchers are convinced that the transdisciplinary lessons drawn from the Yubdo Legabato project have great significance for other mountainous regions in Ethiopia, western Africa, and even the world at large.

THE APPROACH

Community members are no longer considered as simple guinea pigs or data sources. They actively participate in generating knowledge and developing solutions. They become protagonists and change agents. To do so, they must be integrated at all levels of the process — from the initial problem identification, through research and assessment, to the final stage of concrete action. As Mukta Lama, of the Nepalese NGO Social Action for Grassroots Unity and Networking (SAGUN), explains. "We believe that involving people in reflecting on their own situation is the most effective way of raising awareness and internally understanding the need. Through these discussions, community members articulate action plans to address the problems. SAGUN helps them implement such plans and advocates community issues at broader levels."

The way a research project in Buyo, Côte d'Ivoire, was set up offers a good example of the complex negotiating dynamics in the participatory approach. A boom in agricultural production, especially coffee and cocoa, and the building of a hydroelectric dam on the Sassandra River attracted a large number of immigrants to the region. Since 1972, the population has increased from 7 500 to 100 000. The resulting economic, environmental, and social upheaval generated a host of problems, including an indiscriminate use of pesticides and inadequate sanitation.

An Ivorian team set about to improve the situation. From the first preproject workshop that brought together researchers, administrative officials, NGO representatives, village chiefs, men, women, and children, it quickly became clear that the community's concerns were very different from the research team's.

Of course, people wanted to improve the local infrastructure: electricity, roads, clinics, schools, wells, and so on. But what they wanted above all was housing. The construction of the dam had flooded their land and the villagers had been relocated to fibreglass structures. Over a 20-year period, these houses had rotted and were close to collapse. In this environment, it was pointless for the researchers to try to interest the people in the research project: the priority was to address the housing problem. The Ecohealth team therefore contacted local and national authorities. Even though the problem has not yet been completely resolved, the researchers enhanced their credibility by responding to the population's concerns.

Subsequently, the researchers were able to work with the population to address the problem of water contamination. As a result, slow sand filters were installed, which can eliminate 80–90 percent of microbiological contaminants and a large proportion of heavy metals. Their installation was endorsed by a physician from the local hospital, as well as by community members who attended the meetings. Encouraged by these initial successes on the gastro-enteritis front, the community is now expected to move on to other environment-related health problems, such as vector-borne diseases and pesticide exposure.

Increasing participation

Participation by communities in development projects plays out at several levels, ranging from a simple response to researchers' initiatives to taking charge of action programs.

About 95 percent of participatory projects remain at the level of passive participation whereby researchers just tell the people what they plan to do. People then simply provide information and respond to questionnaires. The ecosystem approach to human health, however, aims to achieve at least a level of participation in which people form groups that set concrete goals to improve their environment and health. While most of these groups tend to remain dependent on the outside project initiators, several succeed in becoming autonomous. Other types of participation are even more desirable. One is when communities and researchers jointly participate in an analysis of the problems that leads to action, strengthens existing institutions, and even creates new ones. Such community groups assume responsibility for local decisions. Another level of participation is when communities mobilize to bring about change in their own communities.

Several difficulties and constraints can undermine the implementation of a participatory approach. Levels of participation can vary from one group to the next and need to be negotiated with the partners in each particular context. Every group has its own concerns and interests, which are sometimes compatible with each other but are frequently not. Researchers must therefore demonstrate great care and extraordinary skill in motivating all concerned. An IDRC-supported project with Mapuche indigenous communities in Chile is an example of particularly fruitful community participation (see Box 3, p. 24).

Initially, the tension between the national government and the Mapuches, who were claiming land rights, prevented any collaboration. Considerable internal tension also existed among Mapuche representatives. The research project therefore took these factors into account by immediately working with the Mapuche Association and taking traditional Mapuche knowledge into account in project design.

The researchers and the Mapuche launched a series of workshops to examine the treaties between the Mapuche people and the Chilean government, study Mapuche-related legislation, and review traditional or nontraditional forms of negotiating with the government. Although relations with the Chilean government remain tense, some local Mapuche communities have rekindled a dialogue.

Challenges of the participatory approach

Unfortunately, at this time, very few projects involve communities in the definition of the research question. All too often, researchers continue to consult NGOs, government agencies, and local organizations, while discussions with the people directly concerned are used solely to validate the project.

Many obstacles impede the implementation of a participatory approach. Some communities have had bad experiences with researchers who failed to develop local capacity. A tradition of dependency can also foster the perception that development comes from the outside. Inequalities, power structures, and local elites who hijack the participatory process are other factors that can impede effective community participation.

Other traps await researchers and specialists. Participation should not become a rigid, inflexible ideology: recognizing the value of sharing knowledge should not crystallize into a doctrinal attitude that the local population is always right. The search for new visions, ideas, and values must remain a constant concern. Research team members need to maintain a research-oriented attitude at all times. It is not enough to be the best in one's discipline; it is also necessary to show openness and a genuine desire for collaboration. The participatory approach succeeds when researchers socialize with the local people, stay out of local conflicts, foster the emergence of local leadership, respect all categories of people (including women, children, youth, and the poor), and accept constructive criticism.

However, some objections to this approach persist. For example, opinions differ as to the skill level of local community representatives. Scientists wonder whether local people have sufficient information to participate effectively in defining the research question. Some consider that the local people are not up to the job of describing their health problems in a comprehensible manner to the researchers. No matter: the primary goal is to encourage dialogue between researchers and communities so as to create a common understanding of health problems.

It is often argued as well that local populations do not have the resources to care for their health or to treat illness.

Researchers must clearly explain that the goal is not necessarily to build a hospital or vaccinate children, but to help people identify their own solutions, based on modifications to the ecosystem and resource management. This element is crucial.

In a nutshell, investments in transdisciplinary action and community participation can become the foundations for ensuring that the solutions adopted are sustainable. The resultant improvements in the recipient community's health and environment should repay this investment several times over.

Box 3. | **Improving the Mapuches' quality of life**

The Mapuche indigenous people, now spread out over about half of Argentina and Chile, suffer from serious problems of poverty, poor health, and ecosystem degradation. This deplorable situation is due to in large part to the implementation of policies by leaders who cared little about communicating with indigenous peoples. The goal of one IDRC-supported project in Chile is to find means of managing the ecosystem to provide safe drinking water for the Mapuche living in the Chol Chol valley, 400 km south of Santiago.

The government has converted the Mapuche's ancestral forestlands into large, company-owned farms. These changes have had many harmful consequences: degradation of soils, air, and water; pesticide contamination; loss of biodiversity; food insecurity; and disputes both within and between villages. As a result, the Mapuche have lost all trust in society at large.

Before attempting to change the Mapuche's situation, tensions had to be alleviated: this is what the participatory approach achieved. The Mapuche's views were included in the health program planning process. Several initiatives were launched: a more rational use of pesticides; reintroduction of traditional crops; reforestation with indigenous tree species; adoption of practices that reduce soil erosion; and the establishment of more representative community organizations.

A considerable amount of work still remains to be done to improve relations between municipalities. Survival issues also still loom large. Nonetheless, the people are now better equipped to face these challenges.

Gender and equity

Research does not take place in a vacuum. It is conducted in communities, with men and women whose life is determined by economic, social, and cultural factors. Understanding the qualitative and quantitative differences between the community's various social groups helps to reinforce development action programs.

Gender is one aspect of the Ecohealth approach that sheds light on the way in which male–female relations affect everyone's health. In any community, men and women do things differently. Beyond biology, the gender dimension covers cultural characteristics that define the social behaviour of men and women and the relationships between them. Each gender's particular tasks and responsibilities are constantly being renegotiated in households, workplaces, and communities. This sharing of responsibilities can affect human health, as in the case of communities in northern Côte d'Ivoire.

It is generally assumed that an increase in irrigated rice production results in more cases of malaria, since mosquitoes — the vector of malaria — breed more prolifically in wet environments. However, a comparison of two agroecosystems in northern Côte d'Ivoire, one with no irrigation and one rice harvest per year and the other with irrigation and two harvests per year, has invalidated this hypothesis while confirming the impact of rice culture on the incidence of malaria. There are certainly more mosquitoes and more cases of malaria among young children in the villages with irrigation, but the rate of malaria transmission (the number of infectious bites per year) is identical in both groups.

The IDRC-supported researchers studying this situation postulated that it was not only due to environmental factors, but that social, cultural, and economic factors were also involved. Their research shows that the increase in the number of mosquitoes as a result of irrigation does not necessarily cause an increase in the

Table 1. In villages with two rather than one rice harvest per year, women are more likely to be involved in the harvesting process.

	1 harvest/year	2 harvests/year
Men (primarily)	61%	34%
Women (primarily)	21%	43%
Men and women	18%	23%

Source: de Plaen, R.; Geneau, R. 2002. Cahiers d'études et de recherche francophone/ agriculture, 11(1), 17-22.

transmission of malaria because of the insects' shortened life-span. Rather, the variation in the incidence of malaria between the villages is mainly due to changes in the socioeconomic status of women.

Traditionally in this region, when dry-crop cereals such as millet made up the people's staple diet, family heads were responsible for feeding their families. The moist valley lands were used almost exclusively by women, who would stock the rice and market-garden produce in their personal storehouses. When food was short, the women could use these reserves to help feed their families; they could also sell them to satisfy personal needs or respond to family emergencies (Table 1).

Systematic irrigation of these lands has made it possible to pro-duce two harvests per year, but it has also changed the division of labour. The increase in the quantity of rice grown by women in the valley bottoms has led to a reduction in dry-crop cereals, hitherto grown on the plateaus. Women have thus gradually become responsible for feeding the family. But since the amount of food they can produce is barely adequate to do so, they have little or no opportunity to sell their products in the market. Nor do they have time to participate in additional income-generating agricultural activities. This means they no longer have sufficient income to take quick action at the first signs of illness. Thus, in two-crop villages, women's new status no longer allows then to react as quickly as in villages with only one crop, although, with malaria, early treatment is needed to reduce the severity of an attack. In a nutshell, current levels of malaria are due to more than just biophysical changes in the agroecosystem.

This story well demonstrates the importance of studying all aspects of a problem, and not only its biomedical or environmental dimensions. In the Ecohealth approach, any response or action is useless if differences in gender roles and responsibilities are not taken into account.

Research that takes cultural and socioeconomic differences into account will naturally lead to consideration of the concept of equity. Division of labour is not only a matter of gender; it also varies by social group since people of lower status have access to fewer resources. Consideration of the equity dimension within a gender analysis framework also shows that "male" and "female" are not independent categories, but that the status of individual men and women also depends on their age, ethnic group, and social class. Male–male and female–female differences also exist.

Even though remarkable progress has been made, much still remains to be done to include women and other marginalized groups in the research agenda. For results to be truly convincing, the approach taken needs to be qualitative as well as quantitative, as the problem of battling plague in Tanzania well illustrates.

For almost 20 years, despite constant efforts, plague is still prevalent in the Lushoto region of Tanzania. In fact, it has become virtually endemic. In 1991, an IDRC-supported project called on an epidemiologist and an expert in quantitative social sciences. These two early researchers now work as part of a transdiciplinary team that includes a gender specialist and a specialist in community participation.

Even though the plague problem in Lushoto has not yet been resolved, certain behaviour patterns have been identified that shed new light on the issue. Rural development experts have observed, for instance, that, unlike other communities in eastern

Africa, the residents of Lushoto store their grain stocks under the roofs of their homes, directly above the living quarters. The epidemiologists initially found that women and children were most susceptible to contracting the plague. Anthropologists and other social scientists then discovered the reason: the women and children usually fetch the corn for cooking. They are thus more likely

---

Box 4. | **Healthier farmers in Ecuador**

Carchi province in northern Ecuador is one of the country's main potato producing areas. Here, close to 8 000 farmers grow 40 percent of the national crop.

The use of pesticides and fungicides, which started in the late 1940s, has enabled the people to move from subsistence to cash-crop farming, with a concomitant large increase in family income. However, the rate of pesticide-related deaths in Carchi is one of the highest in the world: 4 people out of 10 000 each year. In the rural areas, 4 percent of the population also suffer from nonlethal poisoning, but do not report their condition to the authorities.

A team of researchers studied three villages using ecosystem approaches to human health: La Libertad, Santa Martha de Cuba, and San Pedro de Piartal. Their transdisciplinary approach included gender-specific parameters. According to an Ecuadorian researcher, the late Veronica Mera-Orcés, the difference between male and female attitudes toward pesticides lies in the fact that "it is widely believed that pesticides cannot harm a strong man." Research has shown, however, that men and women are equally vulnerable: the men are mainly exposed while working in the fields while women and children are in contact with dangerous products either in the houses where the products are stored or when the women wash the men's contaminated clothing.

With the adoption of new, integrated pest-control techniques and better targeted spraying methods, pesticides are now being applied much more efficiently. The result has been a drop of 40–75 percent in the use of certain fungicides and insecticides. Production costs have dropped in tandem, thereby increasing people's income. Now, women are no longer reluctant to tell the men to take care and the men themselves are starting to realize that they should be more careful when handling pesticides.

than adult men to come into contact with the rats infested with plague-bearing fleas that look for food in the same place.

Another specific cultural pattern plays a role in this situation. In large families, nursing women and the men have priority for the household's beds, while children and the other women sleep on the ground where there is a much greater risk of coming into contact with rodents that move around the house at night.

Inclusion of the various social groups in the research agenda is not solely a question of equity; it is, in fact, a question of "good science" to ensure that the research findings are valid. It has even been observed that in social systems subject to a high degree of stress, conflict can often be transformed into cooperation through a strategy that emphasizes women. However, it should also be realized that the increased involvement of women in various committees is itself an additional stressor because of the time and energy they must invest in these tasks.

With its three pillars of transdisciplinarity, participation, and equity, the Ecohealth approach has now proven itself. Communities have changed the ways they manage their environment and have improved their overall health.

Lessons and Successes

The Ecohealth approach has been tested in three major environments that pose serious threats to the health of both ecosystems and people, especially in developing countries: mining, agriculture, and the urban regions.

In each of these sectors, the ecosystem approach to human health has lived up to its potential. And in each can be found the three methodological pillars described in the previous chapter, harbingers of the approach's success and of the identification of concrete, feasible solutions.

Mining

The economy of developing countries depends more than that of most of their industrialized counterparts on the exploitation of natural resources — in fact, that is one way of defining them. In more than 30 developing countries, for instance, mining accounts for 15–50 percent of national exports, while in another 20 it still plays a significant economic role. Small-scale or artisanal mining, most of which is concentrated in the countries of the South, provides work for 13 million people and affects — positively or negatively — the lives of between 80 and 100 million people.

The spectacular growth of mining around the world exerts enormous pressure on ecosytems, which can have harmful repercussions on human health. In Brazil, for instance, the 900 km corridor carved out of the jungle from the Atlantic Ocean to the huge Carajas mine has had an impact on more than 300 000 km^2 of land. The discovery of gold alongside the Tapajos River in Brazil in 1958 provoked a "rush" of some 200 000 prospectors and miners into an undeveloped area totally lacking a sanitary infrastructure.

The life cycle of any mine generally consists of three main phases — exploration and construction, operation, and closure. Each phase presents its particular threats to the health of ecosystems and human populations.

Exploration and construction cause mainly biophysical damage. Low-altitude exploration flights disturb the local people and frighten wildlife. The excavation process causes erosion, makes it easier for pollutants to reach watercourses, and alters animal behaviour patterns. Road-building also leaves scars that often betray the mine's presence in an area. This preliminary phase of a mine's life cycle raises the population's hopes of gainful employment, but it also creates insecurity.

In small-scale and artisanal mines, environmental damage is often due to the high cost of "clean" technologies as well a to a certain indifference on the part of the exploiter. Gold mines, for example, have a number of impacts on the surrounding ecosystem: water is contaminated by metals, vegetation is destroyed, and soil is exposed to erosion. The surrounding communities, for their part, must deal with increased rates of alcoholism, violence, and prostitution. In addition, all types of mines generate potentially dangerous gaseous, liquid, and solid wastes. As a result, many rivers in Africa, Latin America, and Asia have now been declared biologically dead.

Finally, all too often the closing of a mine simply means it is abandoned. It is rare in developing countries for governments to have the means to rehabilitate mines abandoned by the private sector. The situation is even worse in the case of artisanal mines that are often abandoned without any prior planning.

In a mining environment, human health, both physical and mental, is subject to constant assaults. The most common are respiratory irritants, noise pollution, constant vibration, and contaminated drinking water. In many instances, very little is actually known about the various contaminants, their dynamics, and how they are passed to humans. For example, two Ecohealth projects — one dealing with mercury in the Amazon, the other with gold in Ecuador — have shown that the local population's exposure to contaminants does not only come as a result of industrial activity. In fact, agricultural practices such as slash-and-burn cultivation and mountainside cultivation can also release naturally occurring toxins into the environment as a result of soil erosion. This places a double burden on precarious communities, some of which are often located far from the mines.

Mining operations sometimes restrict people's access to arable land, reducing the production of fresh food, and thus harming human health. Local inhabitants also resent the sudden, massive influx of newcomers, precipitated by the opening of new roads: this can lead to conflict. The opening of a mine also affects local women in some countries because they are banned from working in the mines. In several cultures, the presence of a woman in a mine is considered bad luck. This exclusion reduces women's earning potential and thus their influence within both their families and their communities.

The link between the environment and human health is particularly critical in a mining environment. This is why the ecosystem approach to human health, especially through community participation, emerges as a valuable tool for effective action.

Traditionally, studies of the impact of mining on human health and the environment have used a unidisciplinary approach that focuses on a particular issue. For the past 20 years, considerable research has been conducted on environmental pollution, community health, and socioeconomic development. Usually, these specific analyses of particular problems do not make it possible to characterize all facets of a problem in space and time. An enormous gap exists between analysis and effective remedial action.

In countries of the South, conditions in the mines often leave a lot to be desired: the heat, inadequate ventilation, and constant threat of cave-ins create an oppressive working environment for ill-equipped miners, some of whom are very young boys. Wages are low, irregular, and uncertain.

Processing ore also entails its particular share of problems. Miners who use mercury to extract gold often suffer from troubled vision, tremors, and memory loss caused by mercury's toxic effects. Despite the risks for human health and the environment, mercury's ease of use and low cost make it irresistible to gold prospectors. Even small extraction facilities to which miners sometimes bring their ore use techniques that release lead, mercury, manganese, and cyanide into rivers and streams. Within a few years, a charming area recreational area has become a lifeless zone that no one dare use.

In the mining towns of Zaruma and Portovelo in southern Ecuador, IDRC is supporting the Fundación Salud Ambiente y Desarrollo (FUNSAD, an environmental health and development foundation), an NGO that has committed itself to the Ecohealth approach. The foundation has assembled a transdisciplinary team of three doctors, two geologists, a sociologist, and a community development worker. In addition, 12 community members work as project associates, collecting information on the lifestyle and work of 1 800 inhabitants. The third group of key players represent municipal government.

In both cities, people knew that the river was being contaminated by the small ore-processing facilities. They also believed that the water further downstream, below the rapids, was not polluted because of the rapid current. To everyone's surprise, analysis showed the presence of lead many kilometres below the rapids and the processing operations. It seemed impossible for the lead from the factories to be found so far from the mining zones.

Now, it is suspected that lead is released into the environment by land clearing and soil erosion resulting from mountainside cultivation, just as the erosion of the banks of the Amazon's tributaries releases mercury. FUNSAD is also examining atmospheric pollution, especially the effect of climate on pollutant retention in a valley in the heart of the Andean cordillera. In addition, the hypothesis that the lead might come from a contaminated aqueduct has not been eliminated. In addition to these findings and hypotheses, the project has led to talks between the local authorities, the miners, and the communities to find solutions. In southern Ecuador, the transdisciplinary approach has led to the identification of problems that would otherwise have gone unnoticed in a more traditional research context.

Moreover, the use of local people to conduct the interviews proved to be a positive experience. The interviewers did not simply act as sources of data, but involved themselves thoroughly in the process, going so far as to propose solutions. They developed their own vision of the project, including aspects that the researchers had not anticipated, such as controlling the municipality's practice of dumping garbage in the river and implementing an environmental code to reduce the discharge of mining residue into the water. The data-collection team thus transformed itself into a genuine community action group.

This experience shows that the participatory approach works. But the initiative has to germinate within communities and the research team must remain vigilant to ensure that it does not suffocate initiative by adhering at all cost to the project's initial parametres. "What pleases me most in this project," explains Cumanda Lucero, one of the interviewers, "is the feeling of belonging to the community and the hope of being able to improve the situation." FUNSAD's success attests to the principle that "development comes from within."

One of the Ecohealth approach's main challenges in the mining sector is bringing together industry, government, and local community representatives to consult on common problems. Attracted by new legislation in developing countries that throws open the country's doors or by the abundance of mineral resources that can be extracted at very low cost, senior mining companies and a host of junior companies from countries like Australia, Canada, and the United States are investing in new operations. Here as elsewhere, however, each heady period is inevitably followed by a depression. For example, for several years starting in 1993, Latin America experienced a real boom in mining activity that was largely driven by junior firms from Canada.

Since governments in developing countries are often very centralized, local and regional authorities have little power over mining activity. Recent underfinanced efforts at decentralization have faltered, notably because local and regional officials, who have traditionally been excluded from the decision-making process, lack training for their new roles. It is thus difficult, if not impossible, to implement policies formulated further up the hierarchy at the local level, regardless of how enlightened these policies might be.

The situation is complicated by the vulnerability of the populations affected by these new mining activities. Mining stands a

---

Box 5. | **The mines of Goa**

Intensive mining has been underway in Goa for more than 35 years. Because of the employment created and the services provided, the local economy has performed very well indeed. Nevertheless, hillsides have been flattened and forests cleared. People complain of dusty air, dried-up wells, and rain that washes mining waste into rivers, streams, and fields.

A survey of the inhabitants of 57 villages, as well as of mining companies and government representatives, identified common concerns: insufficient compensation for land taken; degradation of air, water, soil, and forests; health problems like diarrhea, jaundice, malaria, flu, and coughs; the eventual closing of the mines; and insufficient investment in recreation, education, and health (Figures 3 and 4).

On the basis of this inventory, a team from the Tata Energy Research Institute of New Delhi identified indicators of well-being and quality of life that all stakeholders accepted. With IDRC assistance, the team succeeded in determining social and environmental performance indicators that, for the first time ever, measured the economic, environmental, and social costs of mining operations. The team also developed optimal revenue criteria to ensure the long-term economic sustainability of mining operations. It can already be stated that the mines' contribution will only be positive if part of their revenues is used to reduce the mines' environmental and social costs for future generations.

These indicators do not solve all the problems, but they do help resolve disputes, make decision-makers more sensitive to everyone's needs and preoccupations, and foster responsibility and transparency. A space for discussion has been created. That's a good start.

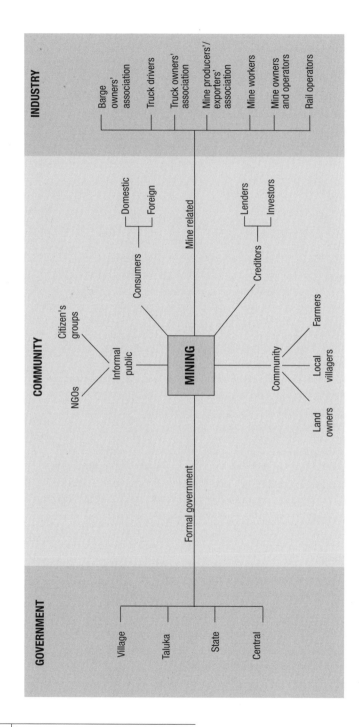

Figure 3.   Stakeholder map for the mining industry in Goa, India (source: Noronha 2001).

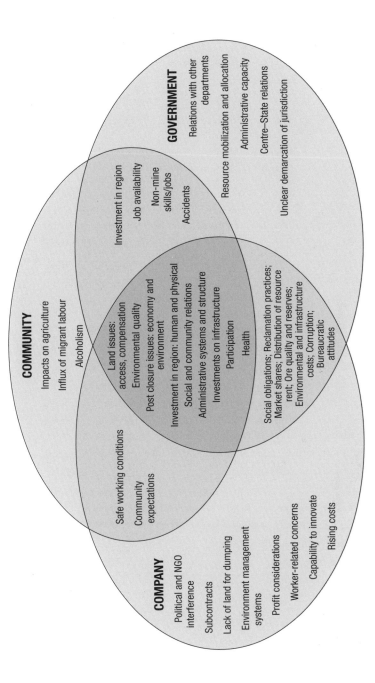

Figure 4. The central intersection shows concerns that are common to the key stakeholders in the Goa mining industry (source: Noronha 2001).

COMMUNITY

Impacts on agriculture
Influx of migrant labour
Alcoholism

GOVERNMENT

Relations with other departments
Resource mobilization and allocation
Administrative capacity
Centre–State relations
Unclear demarcation of jurisdiction

Investment in region
Job availability
Non-mine skills/jobs
Accidents

Land issues: access, compensation
Environmental quality
Post closure issues: economy and environment
Investment in region: human and physical
Social and community relations
Administrative systems and structure
Investments on infrastructure
Participation
Health

Social obligations; Reclamation practices;
Market shares; Distribution of resource
rent; Ore quality and reserves;
Environmental and infrastructure
costs; Corruption;
Bureaucratic
attitudes

Safe working conditions
Community expectations

COMPANY

Political and NGO interference
Subcontracts
Lack of land for dumping
Environment management systems
Profit considerations
Worker-related concerns
Capability to innovate
Rising costs

good chance of aggravating already difficult situations in which poverty, high population densities, and the tropical climate conspire to contaminate the food chain. The need for economic development is great, but a disorganized exploitation of natural resources is likely to deepen poverty. Unfortunately, foreign mining companies have received little training in dealing with social issues in these countries, which are financially so welcoming.

Some companies resist requests for local consultations to avoid costly procedures, especially since mining exploration is always a gamble. Even though some companies are beginning to recognize the importance of local consultation, they do not know how to initiate genuine community participation. A first step would be to include social scientists in mining management teams that until now have almost always been composed solely of geologists and engineers. A further step would be to adopt a transdisciplinary approach.

Moreover, small-scale and artisanal mining operations are booming around the world. They represent a possible way out of poverty for some 13 million untrained workers. But working conditions in these operations remain very hazardous and their impacts on the environment and human health are often devastating.

Governments, communities, and mining companies all face the same problem: a lack of tools for determining the real impact of mining, good and bad, on public health and welfare. Between 1997 and 2002, such tools were developed by a group of scientists from Colombia, India, and the United Kingdom. Specialists from the Tata Energy Research Institute (TERI) in New Delhi, India, then tested these tools in the State of Goa in western India, an area where iron ore has been mined for decades. The Indian team taught the community, the authorities, and the industry how they could use the tools to clearly measure the long-term impact of mining operations on community health and well-being. It would then be up to decision-makers to modify their policies accordingly.

Agriculture

Agricultural production causes profound transformations in the physical and human environment. About 11 percent (1 440 million hectares) of the Earth's land is arable; this area is increasing at the expense of forestland. However, this agricultural land is often poorly managed. For example, excessive use of pesticides and fertilizers, salinization, contamination by heavy metals, and soil depletion have now put about 2 percent of the Earth's lands out of production. This means that more than 10 million hectares of the Earth's arable land have now been irretrievably degraded. Moreover, as pointed out by the WHO in its report entitled *Health and Environment in Sustainable Development* the fluctuations in demand for various agricultural products brings about changes in the ecosystem that affect the health of farmers and their families. Here are some examples, all of which affect the health of both people and ecosystems:

→ Rice is increasingly replacing traditional cereal crops. But the new rice fields are ideal habitats for the vectors of diseases like malaria and schistosomiasis.

→ Changes in the size of livestock herds can, in turn, modify the population densities of biting and blood-sucking insects.

→ The use of new pesticides entails new risks of poisoning.

→ Sometimes, we even go in circles. In Southeast Asia, after deforestation destroyed the habitat of the most important vector of malaria, new plantations of rubber trees, oil palm, and fruit trees recreated even more favourable conditions.

In the agricultural sector, the Ecohealth approach aspires to create synergy between the improvement of agricultural practices and the improvement of human health while ensuring the ongoing viability of agricultural ecosystems.

The Ecohealth approach uses the agroecosystem as the starting point to demonstrate how its judicious management is more

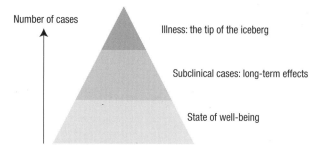

Number of cases

Illness: the tip of the iceberg

Subclinical cases: long-term effects

State of well-being

Figure 5. The health pyramid.

cost-effective in promoting human health than the simple juxta-position of biomedical programs. An "agroecosystem" is simply a coherent geographical and functional entity where agricultural production takes place. Agroecosystems consist of living and non-living components and their interactions. The exact limits of a given agroecosystem are difficult to determine since they depend on the particular question being studied. They can be the bound-aries of a farm, a community, a catchment area, or even an eco-logical region. Dynamic systems, they are affected by factors such as the movement of workers, input of crop seeds and fertilizers, erosion, and seasonal pest infestations. Agroecosystems currently occupy 30 percent of the world's land.

It is not always easy to convince the communities in difficulty that the proposed solution to their health problems is not large-scale vaccination or some other modern medical program, but simply better management of their natural resources. However such an effort is worthwhile, as shown in the health pyramid (Figure 5). Instead of targeting the small fraction of the popula-tion that is severely affected by a given illness — and achieving a very relative success rate — the aim is to attack the root cause of health problems and thereby protect a larger number of people from illness.

Problems linked to pesticides, vector-borne diseases, and malnu-trition abound in countries of the South. The poisoning of farm

Box 6. | Monoculture and health in Kenya

In Kenya, malaria kills between 75 and 100 children every day. Traditional programs to fight this disease have failed. In the Mwea region, the immense tracts of rice paddies that are covered with water six months of the year offer an ideal habitat for mosquitoes. The community has responded with insecticides and antimalarial drugs, but both the mosquitoes and the parasites have become more resistant. Clearly, regardless of cost, another way of dealing with this health problem needs to be found.

After participating in a preproject workshop, a team of specialists from various disciplines launched an Ecohealth study. The team trained 10 villagers as research assistants to interview the inhabitants of four villages on which aspects of their lives they believed were related to malaria.

It was discovered that a very large number of factors have influenced the spread of malaria in Mwea. First, a unique historical and social background has created political conflicts that have affected people's health. Local farmers had recently decided to take responsibility for irrigating their rice fields to escape government control that dated back to the British colonial regime and kept them impoverished. In practice, however, the change has led to agricultural chaos in which farmers plant when and where they want. As a result, the mosquito population and the number of cases of malaria have both increased significantly.

By taking into consideration the many health-related, economic, social, and environmental factors, the villagers and the research team have implemented solutions that improve the environment and do not resort to advanced medical technology. The rice-paddy flooding time has been reduced and the rice crops are now alternated with soybean crops that grow in dry conditions. The mosquitoes' habitat has thus been reduced and people's diet has improved. The children are no longer reduced to eating rice three times a day, a diet that leads to protein deficiency. The families have also been encouraged to surround their houses with plants that repel insects.

One surprising discovery was that the villages with the highest concentrations of mosquitoes were also those with the lowest rates of malaria. But these villages also owned the largest number of cattle. It appears that mosquitoes prefer cattle blood to human blood. That's not to say that increasing herd size would solve the problem, however. Strains of bacteria that kill mosquito larvae but are harmless to humans have been introduced into the water. It was also recommended that women and children — the more vulnerable members of the population — sleep under insecticide-treated mosquito nets.

The researchers have established a genuine relationship with the communities. The villagers now have greater self-confidence since they have realized that they can act effectively on their environment and improve their health.

With support from the International Water Management Institute, scientists and representatives from NGOs, government, and the communities are now working to disseminate the Mwea experience throughout Kenya. Through a framework called the System-Wide Initiative on Malaria and Agriculture (SIMA), they are institutionalizing the Ecohealth approach. The initiative's goal is to put in place ways of reducing malaria while improving people's health and increasing agricultural productivity. This program provides a research and development framework that generates practical short-term solutions while responding to the needs of targeted communities in both the medium and long term. The establishment of SIMA ensures the sustainability of the Ecohealth approach in Kenya.

labourers, the explosive increase in the number of malaria cases from the digging of irrigation canals, and the impact of mono-cultural food production on the quality of people's diets — all are striking examples of crucial problems that can be addressed using an approach that takes the link between ecosystem and human health into account.

The Ecohealth approach has already borne fruit in situations involving each of these problems. In the Mwea region of Kenya, better control of the malaria-carrying mosquito has been achieved by modifying agricultural practices (Box 6). In Oaxaca, Mexico, deliberations involving scientists, community groups, and government decision-makers have led to the introduction of community actions that have essentially wiped out the region's use of DDT (Box 7). In the highlands of Yubdo Legabato, Ethiopia, extensive community involvement has enabled the local population to break the vicious cycle of poverty and malnutrition (see Box 2, p. 19).

Box 7. | An end to DDT use in Mexico

In Mexico in the 1940s and 1950s, close to 24 000 of the 2.4 million people who caught malaria every year died as a result. Massive use of the powerful insecticide DDT was the linchpin of the government's effort to eradicate the disease. Over time, some progress was made against malaria, but the war was far from won. The use of DDT also posed its own threats to the health of the ecosystem. Moreover, as required by the North American Free Trade Agreement, Mexico had to completely eliminate the use of DDT by 2002.

To meet this challenge, an Ecohealth research project was set up to pool the knowledge of a team of specialists in epidemiology, computer science, entomology, and social sciences, from both government and academia.

This team has accumulated volumes of information about the prevalence of malaria in 2 000 villages. Data from powerful geographical information systems enabled them to conclude that mosquitoes do not travel very much. "If you have a place to lay your eggs and feed yourself, why go elsewhere?" explains Mario Henry Rodriguez, Director of Research on Infectious Diseases at the National Institute for Public Health (NIPH). In addition, as confirmed by Juan Eugenio Hernández, NIPH's Director of Informatics, it is now believed that "human beings are the vectors of malaria," which explains why more cases of malaria are found in villages located alongside roads.

With community help, the team studied the population's living conditions, including behavioural differences between men and women. It was found that while women are more likely to be bitten by mosquitoes early in the morning when they go to fetch water, the men are likely to be bitten in the coffee plantations at night.

Several preventive actions have been taken. The scientists have proposed a new insecticide that, unlike DDT, does not persist in the environment. They have also developed a more effective pump that can spray 40 homes a day instead of 8, and uses less insecticide. A new malaria testing kit now detects the presence or absence of parasites in a patient's blood in only a few minutes, unlike laboratory tests that take three to four weeks to confirm a diagnosis. Previously, the need to wait for test results forced the authorities to treat everyone who showed vague symptoms of the illness, such as a high fever or headaches. Now, volunteers administer these tests to the people in close to 60 villages. "We have given communities the means to take care of themselves," says Mario Rodriguez.

CASE STUDIES

The fight against malaria in Mexico is now no longer solely the responsibility of government employees. Women also play a role by removing, every two weeks, the algae that harbour mosquito larvae in bodies of water. As a result, the number of cases of malaria in the state of Oaxaca has dropped from 15 000 in 1998 to only 400 today — and all without using any DDT. "Our experience has taught us that we need to bolster the social science research component if we want to extend this program to other parts of the country, while maintaining it in Oaxaca. The challenge is to draw the lessons that will lead to application of the program on a much wider scale," says Dr Rodriguez.

Most of these successful actions are not new. Their effectiveness is, however, in large part due to the adoption of a transdisciplinary approach in identifying problems and applying various solutions.

The urban environment

At the current rate of urban growth, every year the Earth will welcome one new 10-million-resident megacity and about 10 other million-plus cities. In fact, most of the world's 6.3 billion people live in cities or their immediate vicinity. In developing countries, cities face immense and disheartening challenges. One hundred million newcomers flock to cities each year, many of them rural people in search of better living conditions.

In the ecosystem approach to human health, the urban environment is characterized as an ecosystem that is largely influenced by human activity. Its distinctive features are high population density, an established infrastructure, and a high level of social organization. Cities offer very specific challenges for the Eco-health approach. Researchers studying human health and the environment in an urban setting need to be concerned about poverty, housing, security, human rights, and equity.

Until now, IDRC-supported urban Ecohealth projects have mainly dealt with capitals — Kathmandu in Nepal, Mexico City in Mexico, and Havana in Cuba — in addition to one project in the city of Buyo, Côte d'Ivoire. In these large agglomerations, many groups with diverse interests interact: the private sector, civil society, municipal authorities, different ethnic groups, castes, and social classes, men and women. All play a role in the management of the urban ecosystem. This complicates the implementation of effective remedial programs, as shown by an air pollution reduction project in Mexico City.

The air in Mexico City, situated 2 240 m above sea level in a large valley, often contains two to three times more pollutants than international standards deem acceptable. Launched in 2000, the 10-year PROAIRE program seeks to improve air quality sufficiently to reduce the rate of pollution-related illness and deaths. From the outset, it has taken for granted that the inhabitants of the world's largest megacity will need to change their living habits. Achieving this, however, first requires understanding clearly how the residents perceive the air pollution problem.

With this goal in mind, federal authorities called on several national and international organizations, including women's groups and other organizations concerned with health and the environment, to clearly identify the problem and develop actions to solve it. In a city as large as Mexico, it can be difficult to motivate people to act. Thus, in addition to determining people's perceptions of the causes and effects of air pollution, researchers also sought to determine what, if any, action they were willing to take to fight it.

The survey revealed a tendency to blame air pollution on factories. Only a few of respondents mentioned the role of car exhaust, which actually accounts for 75 percent of all harmful emissions. People say "Other people are mainly responsible: my neighbours, maybe, but not me, not my car. My family and lifestyle are not to blame," reports Roberto Muñoz of the Secretaria del Medio Ambiente, the organization that directed this IDRC-funded project. Most people admit to not taking any action to deal with air pollution, nor are they interested in participating in air-improvement programs. The government, they say, is in a better position to deal with the situation than they are.

To convince people of their responsibilities and their ability to improve the situation, community education programs were required. The researchers found that past government programs had been largely ineffective. To formulate effective approaches, 14 workshops, each consisting of 8–21 participants (homemakers, local leaders, and so on), were organized in six separate districts of the city. Together, researchers and community members developed training materials and programs that educate people not only about the scale of Mexico City's problem but also about concrete actions men and women can take in the home and community to help solve it — for example, using public transportation and carpooling, reducing water and fuel consumption, and using organic products.

Because cities are social organizations that evolve very rapidly, both spatially and socially, community participation becomes all the more difficult to maintain. One effective way of promoting participation has been to target smaller communities within the city itself. In Mexico City, six districts were chosen to organize workshops. In Kathmandu, after consulting men and women from different castes, two neighbourhoods were chosen in which the key players and environmental factors harmful to human health had been accurately identified. In Cuba, it is the residents of a small Havana neighbourhood, Cayo Hueso, who have come together to find solutions to the problems of housing and poverty that affect their health.

In 1995, the inhabitants of Cayo Hueso decided to rehabilitate their historic neighbourhood: fewer than half the residents had access to drinking water, more than a third of the living quarters

Box 8. | Cleaning up Kathmandu, Nepal

Kathmandu, the capital of Nepal, is currently experiencing one of the fastest population growth rates in South Asia. The process of urbanization there has been speeding up since 1950 and is characterized by both modernization and under-development. In Kathmandu, a wealthy elite rubs shoulders more or less comfortably with poor people belonging to lower castes and ethnic minorities.

Between 1998 and 2001, an IDRC-funded Ecohealth research project led to a better understanding of the dynamics between the various sociocultural, economic, political, and environmental determinants of human health. Two Nepalese NGOs played a key role in this project: one focused on diseases that humans share with animals; the other concentrated on sociocultural aspects and community participation strategies.

In the two wards of the city chosen for the project, 57 different castes live and work side by side — among them priests, peasants, artisans, butchers, street-sweepers, and hairdressers. The traditions imported from the countryside vary widely and are often incompatible with sustainable urban development. In the neighbourhoods studied, for example, 87 percent of households usually throw their wastes directly onto the street rather than into garbage bins. The street-sweepers, most of them women accompanied by their children, are responsible for managing the solid waste. Moreover, 96 percent of the butchers were not aware of the contamination dangers posed by meat wastes, and their butchering techniques facilitated the transmission of animal diseases to humans.

The organizations taking part in the projects have helped the government regulate animal slaughtering: it is no longer permitted to slaughter animals on the banks of the Bishnumati River or to use its water to clean dead animals. The government has also helped an entire population of homeless immigrants organize literacy classes and look after their own primary health care needs, except for cases that actually require a physician's attention.

The Kathmandu urban system turned out to be much more complex than originally imagined and the project clearly showed the importance of planning and acting in concert with onsite organizations. Dr D.D. Joshi, Director of Nepal's National Zoonoses and Food Hygiene Research Centre, believes that this project owes its success to a marriage of science and awareness of social dynamics, which the Ecohealth approach facilitated.

CASE STUDIES

had been declared unhealthy, and infections like tuberculosis and sexually transmitted diseases were on the rise. Through a community organization called Taller Integral (integral workshop) the community channelled its efforts and those government organizations. "In this part of Cuba," says Mariano Bonet, leader of the IDRC-funded Ecohealth project, "scientists and the people are already closely connected because researchers from the country's National Institute of Hygiene, Epidemiology, and Microbiology, the main vehicle for government involvement, actually live in the area."

The government has invested in restoring the district's buildings and has improved the water supply and garbage disposal systems. Special areas have been built for young people and street lighting has been improved. "One of the challenges," adds Mariano Bonet, "has been to translate the technical aspects of the research into language that the community can easily understand, as well as to convert community expertise into indicators and specific activities."

In the end, people from all walks of life participated in the project, including older women who made sandwiches. These first efforts have led to better social planning, including programs for seniors that involve activities such as physical exercise sessions and self-esteem workshops.

Scientists monitor the complex interactions between the urban fabric and the population's health. For example, for the first time ever, a study has been carried out of the connections between people's quality of life and specific factors like street lighting, water availability, and garbage collection. These studies have been carried out by a team composed of doctors, engineers, a sociologist, a psychologist, an economist, and an architect. A comparison of the health of the residents of Cayo Hueso with that of the residents in another community that had not benefited from similar interventions revealed a definite improvement in the health of Cayo Hueso's teenagers, adult men, and older women. Equally significant: in the wake of this program, a woman now chairs the people's council of Cayo Hueso.

Because of the exemplary success of the Cayo Hueso program, IDRC is now funding Dr Bonet's team in a project to control dengue fever, a pressing health problem in Latin America and Asia that is closely linked to the environment.

In Côte d'Ivoire, Cuba, Mexico, and Nepal, women's associations have been integrated into the definition of the research question. Interestingly it appears that urban women organize themselves and defend their rights better than their rural sisters. To truly respect the principle of male–female equity, it is important to recognize men's and women's distinct roles and responsibilities and understand how each gender is affected differently. This principle also needs to be extended to all groups when necessary, as was the case in Kathmandu where rich and poor — such as the untouchable street-sweepers — live and work side by side.

Researchers funded by IDRC are now developing indicators that will make it possible to evaluate the progress achieved toward sustainable development and better human health in the cities. Although generic indicators have existed for many years, indicators better suited to the unique characteristics of individual projects are needed. In Cuba, for example, it has already been shown that certain indicators such as the incidence of asthma, the presence of street lighting, and the rate of economic and urban growth very much reflect the environment's health in relation to the health of its human inhabitants.

Comprehensible results, sustainable solutions

One of the most notable successes of the ecosystem approach to human health, as promoted by IDRC, occurred in the Amazon where it was discovered that soil erosion was the main cause of mercury contamination. The Ecohealth approach has also made

Box 9. | Mercury in the Amazon

In the mid-1980s, Brazilian physician and cardiologist Fernando Branches alerted the scientific community that one of his patients, whom he believed was suffering from heart problems, had actually been poisoned by mercury. In short order, several international research teams became interested in the problem. In 1995, an IDRC-funded team consisting of researchers from the Federal University of Para in Belem, Brazil, the Federal University of Rio de Janeiro, and the Université du Québec à Montréal (UQAM) made an astonishing discovery — the mercury contamination believed to be due to traditional mining operations was actually much more closely linked to certain farming practices.

Since the 1970s, a genuine gold rush has taken place along the banks of the Tapajos River, a major tributary of the Amazon. The artisanal method used to extract the gold employs mercury: when the metal comes into contact with gold it causes it to melt and amalgamate. Easily recovered, this amalgam is then heated. The mercury evaporates, leaving behind the prospector's glittering reward.

The Canadian researchers and their Brazilian counterparts expected to see the level of mercury in the water decrease the further they moved away from the mining area. Surprisingly, however, the concentration in the water remained the same up to 400 km from the mining site. This clearly indicated that something other than mines was the source of mercury contamination.

From time immemorial, volcanoes have been spewing mercury, which eventually falls to the ground. More recently, industrial activity like waste incineration has also contributed. It is estimated that the very old soils in the Amazon basin have been accumulating mercury for 500 000 to one million years, but this mercury has remained locked up in the soil until recent times. Since the 1950s, new settlers, attracted by the availability of farm land, have cut down and burned more than 2.5 million hectares of Amazon forest, mainly along the rivers. The rain falling directly onto the soil has been washing the mercury into the rivers, where bacteria convert it into toxic methyl mercury. The bacteria then pass the methyl mercury onto smaller fish, which are then eaten by bigger fish that eventually end up in people's frying pans. Terminal predators, humans thus absorb the highest concentrations of mercury.

The Brazilian and Canadian researchers demonstrated that even though the mercury levels in the hair of the villagers taking part in the study were well within WHO standards, they showed signs of a loss of coordination, manual dexterity, and visual acuity.

It appeared that the quantity of methyl mercury in people's bodies was linked to their consumption of different types of fish, which varied from season to season. People who ate herbivorous fish were less affected than those who ate carnivorous fish, which contained the highest mercury levels.

The second stage of the project consisted of working with the villagers to find solutions. A close working relationship with village women as well as with local teachers, health workers, and fisherfolk was established. One of the results of this collaboration has been a poster, suggested by the community, that shows the various types of fish and their level of contamination. It is now common knowledge that it is better to "eat fish that do not eat other fish." The results are very concrete: between 1995 and 2002, mercury concentrations in the villagers' hair have dropped by 40 percent (Figure 6).

For several months, midwives kept an exact record of the food eaten by 30 village women. It was also discovered by analyzing segments of their hair — each of which represents one month's growth — that mercury levels were lower in women who ate more fruit. This led to identifying foods that are likely to lower mercury levels in the human body.

The villagers have also started to change their farming practices. Working together, researchers and local farmers identified crops that could improve people's diet while reducing the likelihood of further mercury leaching. The researchers have also worked with local fisherfolk to locate the sections of the river that are least conducive to the transformation of mercury into its toxic derivative, methyl mercury.

In collaboration with the people living alongside the Tapajos River, research is continuing to apply scientific findings to their lives and thereby improve their health and that of their environment.

it possible to test various short- and medium-term strategies that have already reduced the level of human poisoning. The great advantage of the Ecohealth method was confirmed by better community health.

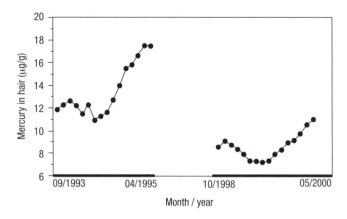

Figure 6. From 1995 to 2002 levels of mercury in the hair of people living by the Tapajos River dropped by 40 percent. (Source: Mergler, D., personal communication, 2003)

During the project, the research team learned — sometimes the hard way — how to interact with local communities, then attract the interest of local decision-makers. Initially intuitive, this process developed and evolved because of the trust established between the partners. The input of new expertise, especially in the social sciences, as the research proceeded, played a crucial role. The challenge of how to involve decision-makers in the research process remains, but dialogue has been opened and the partners are actively looking for agricultural development alternatives for the region.

It was initially difficult to interest the local authorities in the project because they were not involved when it was launched. It must be recalled that the project was not transdisciplinary at the outset: fieldwork and the needs felt by the partners oriented its evolution. This clearly shows the pioneering role this team has played in introducing the Ecohealth research framework within IDRC.

The formulation and understanding of this particular problem evolved over time: even after 10 years there is room for improvement. During this period, many Canadian and Brazilian students were trained in the field and obtained their master's or doctoral degree. Currently, four Brazilian researchers are pursuing their doctorates on project-related topics. This has been one of the project's great successes: in addition to changes in environmental management and health care practices in the area, there is now a new generation of scientists to continue the work.

Before the arrival of the IDRC-funded team, several teams from Japan, Europe, and other parts of the world had worked in the project site but, despite their scientific competence, had failed to bring about any real change. In the IDRC-funded project, the ecosystem approach to human health led to improvements in the community's health as early as the third year, partly because of a change in the type of fish eaten.

In most countries where communities and groundbreaking teams have tried the Ecohealth approach, processes to improve environmental and human health have arisen. One of the main challenges then becomes how to apply the results on a larger scale.

Chapter 4

Recommendations and Future Directions

A community of Canadian and international scientists and decision-makers is beginning to appreciate the Ecohealth approach. It is also gaining followers in the research and educational communities, as well as among policymakers, who are learning about it in various ways.

Early recognition

In March 2002, at the first meeting of environment and health ministers of the Americas, held in Ottawa, Canada, Mexico's health minister, Julio Frenk, spoke about the success of the Ecohealth approach in solving the dilemma of DDT as a malaria-control agent in Mexico (see Box 7, p. 45). In Johannesburg in

August 2002, Canadian Minister of the Environment David Anderson took up the torch and stressed the pertinence of examining the links between the environment and human health. "The challenge for decision-makers," said Mr. Anderson, "is that too often we only have a very general idea of the links between health and the environment. We have to ensure that government departments coordinate their efforts." He closed by pointing to the importance of the International Forum on Ecosystem Approaches to Human Health in Montréal in May 2003 as an example of an initiative that "will help us reach and share our goals in the health and environment fields."

The Ecohealth approach is also gradually gaining ground in the scientific community. Here are some examples:

➤ The approach was presented at a panel on research, health, and development jointly organized by IDRC and the US National Institutes of Health (NIH) at the World Summit on Sustainable Development, in Johannesburg, in August 2002.

➤ It has been adopted by the Special Programmme for Research and Training in Tropical Diseases (TDR), an independent collaborative program cofunded by the United Nations Development Programme, the World Bank, and WHO. With IDRC support, TDR is applying the Ecohealth approach in two research programs in South America.

➤ In addition, the Pan American Health Organization is providing technical support for the implementation of the approach in two dengue fever projects in Central America and the Caribbean. These projects are also supported by the United Nations Environment Programme (UNEP).

Ecosystem approaches to human health are also being increasingly adopted by educational institutions:

➤ In August 2002, Mexico's Instituto Nacional de Salud Publica offered a summer course on the Ecohealth approach, attended by some 30 people.

➤ The American University of Beirut has set up a graduate inter-faculty program in environmental sciences that includes the Ecohealth approach.

➤ In Canada, the University of Guelph, the Institute of Environmental Sciences at UQAM, the faculties of medicine and dentistry at the University of Western Ontario, and various other institutions active in the interplay between health and the environment now offer this type of program.

The establishment of such programs provides hope for researchers who have ventured in this new direction: they are proof that institutions are changing and that there will be space for them and their students.

In addition, a national consultation on the future of transdisciplinary programs in health and the environment, overseen by the Canadian Institutes of Health Research, underscored the innovative character of the Ecohealth approach. In Canada, the Ecohealth approach is "coming out of the scientific closet:" it is being presented to the public at scientific exhibitions, as well as in pamphlets and popular science articles.

Finally, interest in the ecosystem approaches to human health is confirmed by the International Forum on Ecosystem Approaches to Human Health, held in Montréal, May 18–26, 2003. WHO, UNEP, the Ford Foundation, the United Nations Foundation, the Canadian International Development Agency, the Canadian ministries of health and environment, the Québec Ministry of Health and Social Services, UQAM, and the Montréal Biodôme have supported its organization. This forum confirms the existence of an international "Ecohealth approach" community: this forum is its first international meeting.

Challenging scientists

Above all, the Ecohealth approach requires the application of its three methodological pillars: transdisciplinarity, community participation, and gender sensitivity. This does not imply rejecting disciplinary research, which remains essential: each researcher must conserve his or her identity. A delicate balance also needs to be maintained between community needs and the interests of decision-makers and scientists.

Defining a common language calls for a major effort from all concerned. It implies real risks for researchers even within their own institutions since it requires deviating from predetermined research areas and demands a sustained effort. It can lead to delayed publications and uncertain interactions with local people. Finally, it requires learning how civil and political structures operate. In this context, educational institutions must accept the risks by providing the needed resources and assessing results in ways other than simply counting the number of publications generated. These institutions need to allow their academic departments to collaborate beyond multidisciplinarity.

Challenges for decision-makers

At a later stage, the Ecohealth approach will need to see its project results incorporated into larger scale programs and policies. This will require that policymakers well understand the issues and methods associated with this approach. They will need to go beyond the superficial, become full participants in sustainable development, articulate their needs, and, above all, be patient. They will also need to be genuinely interested in the work of the researchers.

Acknowledging that the study of complex problems is a lengthy process is key to the approach's success. For instance, it can take two or three years to set up a trandisciplinary team and define a common language, although this timeframe has been reduced to one year in some recent projects. An encouraging aspect, however, is that the ecosystem approach to human health produces results throughout the project's life, making it possible to take continuous action to improve the health of the community and the environment.

Financial support clearly plays a crucial role. If it is withdrawn during the course of the project, the project simply disappears. Because the continuation of a project is very much dependent on its funding, researchers whose parent institutions do not accept and support the Ecohealth approach are treading on dangerous ground.

The promise of the Ecohealth approach

For municipal, regional, and national decision-makers struggling with situations in which the environment affects human health, the ecosystem approach to human health provides a readily applicable process that can also point the way toward viable long-term solutions.

Decision-makers need practical, adequate, inexpensive, and feasible solutions. The quest for such solutions is at the heart of Ecohealth methodology. Ecohealth teams do not see their task as simply accumulating data; they are continually motivated to find solutions. "Of course, we can study problems," says Dr Oscar Betancourt, director of Ecuador's FUNSAD NGO, "but studies are simply studies." From the outset, Ecohealth projects work toward identifying practical solutions. "It's a technique for finding solutions, not just for describing problems," adds Dr David Waltner-Toews of the University of Guelph in Canada, who is also working to develop research methods that focus on the links between the environment and human health.

For policymakers, the Ecohealth approach offers many potentially important advantages. It allows public servants from various ministries to work together around a common scientific core with groups having different or opposing interests. In Mexico, public servants and other government officials who put Ecohealth principles into practice in the fight against malaria have concluded that it is the right approach. This Ecohealth project has created a negotiated space in which representatives from disparate ministries, departments, and disciplines (agriculture, environment, health) work together. Guided and motivated by a common search for solutions, they can set aside their differences to concentrate on their particular contribution to the problem's solution.

The same is true for various citizens' organizations with clearly defined and sometimes divergent interests. For them also, the project creates a space where they can work together. In some cases, groups that are otherwise in conflict work side by side. In some communities, the project offers a forum for discussion among representatives of business, citizen groups, and government organizations. It can even happen, as in Kathmandu, that the project stimulates dialogue between representatives of castes separated by centuries of contempt.

Ecohealth projects usually begin with an alliance between scientists and community members. These alliances find themselves greatly strengthened when decision-makers agree to participate. Government authorities need to understand that the participation of public servants in such projects is necessary. They also must accept that their staff operate in a new framework characterized by transdisciplinarity, community participation, and social equity. In practice, the initiative can come from any of the partners. Even national authorities, as in Mexico, have launched such projects.

The Ecohealth approach offers a place at the table for representatives of any agency, jurisdiction, or authority interested in helping to improve a situation. Decision-makers are provided with integrated solutions that take into account the various actors, including those over which they exercise direct authority (public servants) and those over which they don't (citizens' groups). When completed, a project can even result in the creation of a new managerial entity, as in the case of southern Ecuador where a new body now represents two communities affected by mining waste. Since representatives of the relevant policymaking authorities are already acquainted with each other and there is eventual consensus on solutions, it becomes easier to harmonize policies — always a challenge for mayors, governors, and ministers. The program can then be adjusted in response to the needs and new solutions identified during the research.

In the wake of an Ecohealth project in Kenya, a program was launched to study the application of the Ecohealth approach to several communities in that country. As well, the mercury project in the Amazon basin has now had ramifications in Canada. In 2001, the Natural Sciences and Engineering Research Council of Canada (NSERC) supported the creation of COMERN, the Collaborative Mercury Research Network. The network connects researchers from across Canada who are concerned with the safe and sustainable use of our aquatic resources, with a focus on the problems posed by mercury contamination (Figure 7). The integrated ecosystem approach advocated by COMERN includes the active participation of specialists in all fields of the applied sciences, as well as social interveners and political decision-makers in all steps of research development. Many of the Canadian researchers in the network, including the coordinator Dr Marc Lucotte, are also associated with the Amazon project.

Use of the Ecohealth approach immediately sets in motion a collaborative process whereby all the key players come together around the same table to produce applicable and feasible long-term solutions. Of course, this means taking the risk of placing confidence in a disparate team, investing the time and resources required, and the will to change things.

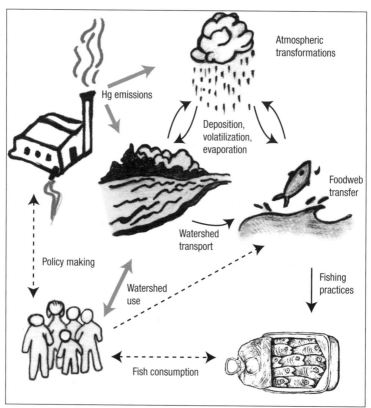

Figure 7. COMERN, the Collaborative Mercury Research Network, uses the ecosystem approach to study the movement of mercury through the environment in Canada. (Source: Lucotte, M., personal communication, 2003)

One of the reasons for the success of the Ecohealth approach is that the proposed solutions take into account local knowledge and the contribution of community members. For example, women from the villages along the Tapajos River in Brazil have spread the word about the species of fish that are less contaminated and therefore safe to eat. In the South, communities are often left to fend for themselves. But if "experts" arrive to study their problems, the Ecohealth methodology creates a space in which decision-makers, community members, and researchers can combine forces.

Accepting that it is their responsibility to change a situation is generally facilitated when people have participated in defining the problem. In Ethiopia, for instance, once the villagers that were the focus of an Ecohealth project realized that their sanitation practices were affecting their health, they took the situation in hand.

Decision-makers obtain a menu of solutions in an area that both families and individuals regard as priority — their health. The solutions advocated do not deal only with changes in behaviour. They also bear on better understanding the interactions between environmental, social, economic, and political aspects of the problem to be solved. They ensure that the eventual investments in infrastructure and new services will be made in the right places, and in places where people can see immediate results. What's more, the relatively short lapse of time between initiating the process and the first visible results makes it easier to implement longer term interventions.

Of course, when authorities support Ecohealth projects, as described in this small book, they take certain risks — but one of those risks is success! In Brazil, Cuba, Mexico, Nepal, and a growing number of other countries, success has been achieved. But before launching an Ecohealth project, make sure that there is a leader, supported by his or her institution or community. These leaders exist: they are the driving force of the Ecohealth approach. Increasingly, they are found in research environments, in remedial action programs, and in government policymaking.

For some of them, the Ecohealth approach has already brought prizes, promotions, and recognition. In Mexico, for example, the leader of the Ecohealth project received the prestigious Jorge Rosenkranz Award in 2002. In Cuba, the project leader was given the Cuban Academy of Sciences' Health Award, one of the country's highest scientific distinctions. By encouraging Ecohealth projects, government authorities who successfully associate themselves with the work of researchers and communities make winners out of everyone.

The current results of the ecosystem approach to human health represent a few concrete answers to the challenges of sustainable development. They also provide reason to hope.

Sources and Resources

This book focuses on the research that IDRC has supported on ecosystem approaches to human health, or Ecohealth. For those interested in learning more about Ecohealth in general, there is a great deal of published literature, both in print and on the Internet. This appendix offers a selection of resources for further study. The list is structured in roughly the same way as the book, providing resources for each chapter.

This book also forms an integral part of IDRC's Ecohealth Web site **www.idrc.ca/ecohealth**. The full text of the book is available online and leads the reader into a virtual web of resources, including many of those listed here.

The Issue

For a useful general overview of ecosystem approaches to human health, including background and various methodologies, tools, and case studies, the following publications are recommended:

Forget, D. 2003. Jean Lebel: penser globalement, agir localement. Découvrir, mars–avril 2003. Association francophone pour le savoir, Montréal, QC, Canada.

Forget, G.; Lebel, J. 2001. An ecosystem approach to human health. International Journal of Occupational and Environmental Health, 7(2), S1–S38.

Forget, G.; Lebel, J. 2003, Approche écosystémique à la santé humaine. *In* Gérin, M.; Gosselin, P.; Cordier, S.; Viau, C.; Quénel, P.; Dewailly, É., ed., Environnement et santé publique: fondements et pratiques. Diffusion and Edisem, St Hyacinthe, QC, Canada. Chapter 23, pp. 593–640.

Lebel, J.; Burley, L. 2003. The ecosystem approach to human health in the context of mining in the developing world. *In* Rapport, D.J.; Lasley, W.L.; Rolston, D.E.; Nielsen, N.O.; Qualset, C.O.; Damania, A.B., ed., Managing for healthy ecosystems. Lewis Publishers, Boca Raton, FL, USA. Chapter 83, pp. 819–834.

Smit, B.; Waltner-Toews, D.; Rapport, D.; Wall, E.; Wichert, G.; Gwyn, E.; Wandel, J. 1998. Agroecosystem health: analysis and assessment. University of Guelph, Guelph, ON, Canada.

Waltner-Toews, D. 1996. Ecosystem health: a framework for implementing sustainability in agriculture. Bioscience, 46, 686–689

The following documents and events are mentioned or referred to in this book:

Agenda 21: **http://www.un.org/esa/sustdev/documents/ agenda21/index.htm**

Comité d'études sur la promotion de la santé. 1984. Objectif santé : rapport du comité d'étude sur la promotion de la santé. Conseil des affaires sociales et de la famille, Gouvernement du Québec, Québec, Canada.

CPHA (Canadian Public Health Association). 1992. Human health and the ecosystem: Canadian perspectives, Canadian action. CPHA, Ottawa, ON, Canada.

Epp, J. 1986. Health for all. Health and Welfare Canada, Ottawa, ON, Canada.

Forget, G. 1997. From environmental health to health and the environment: research that focuses on people. *In* Shahi, G.S.; Levy, B.S.; Binger, A.; Kjellström, T.; Lawrence, R., ed., International perspectives on environment, development and health: toward a sustainable world. Springer, New York, NY, USA. pp. 644–659.

Hancock, T. 1990. Toward healthy and sustainable communities: health, environment and economy at the local level. Paper presented at the 3rd Colloquium on Environmental Health, Québec, Canada, 22 November 1990.

ILRI (International Livestock Research Institute). 2001. Enhanced human well-being through livestock/natural resource management: final technical report to IDRC. ILRI, Addis Ababa, Ethiopia.

International Forum on Ecosystem Approaches to Human Health: **www.idrc.ca/forum2003**

Lalonde, M. 1974. A new perspective on the health of Canadians: working paper. Government of Canada, Ottawa, ON, Canada.

Lucotte, M. 2000. Collaborative research network program on the impacts of atmospheric mercury deposition on large-scale ecosystems in Canada: the COMERN Initiative — Research Network Proposal to NSERC. Natural Sciences and Engineering Council of Canada, Ottawa, ON, Canada.

Mining, Minerals and Sustainable Development (MMSD) Project. 2002. Breaking new ground: mining, minerals and sustainable development. Earthscan, London, UK. **www.iied.org/mmsd/ finalreport/index.html**

Report of the United Nations Conference on the Human Environment (Stockholm 1972): **www.unep.org/Documents/ Default.asp?DocumentID=97**

Rio Declaration on Environment and Development: **www.un.org/ documents/ga/conf151/aconf15126-1annex1.htm**

Tansley, A.G. 1935. The use and misuse of vegetational terms and concepts. Ecology, 16, 284–307.

United Nations Environment Programme. 2002. Global environmental outlook 3 (GEO3). Earthscan, London, UK, **www.unep.org/GEO/geo3/**

WHO (World Health Organization). 1998. Health and environment in sustainable development: five years after the Earth Summit. WHO, Geneva, Switzerland. **www.who.int/archives/ inf-pr-1997/en/pr97-47.html**

World Commission on Environment and Development. 1987. Our common future. Oxford University Press, Oxford, UK.

World Summit on Sustainable Development: **www.johannesburgsummit.org**

The Approaches, Lessons, and Successes

Key references and Web sites related to the projects presented in these chapters are listed below. All of these projects have submitted detailed interim or final technical reports, many of which can be found online at **www.idrc.ca/ecohealth** or requested by contacting **ecohealth@idrc.ca**.

Mercury Exposure, Ecosystem, and Human Health in the Amazon

This long-running series of projects is featured at **www.facome.uqam.ca** and has produced the following publications:

Amorim, M.I.; Mergler, D.; Bahia, M.O.; Dubeau, H.; Miranda, D.; Lebel, J.; Burbano, R.R.; Lucotte, M. 2000. Cytogenetic damage related to low levels of methyl mercury contamination in the Brazilian Amazon. An. Acad. Bras. Cienc., 72(4), 497–507.

Dolbec, J.; Mergler, D.; Larribe, F.; Roulet, M.; Lebel, J.; Lucotte, M. 2001. Sequential analysis of hair mercury levels in relation to fish diet of an Amazonian population, Brazil. The Science of Total Environment, 271(1-3), 87–97.

Dolbec, J.; Mergler, D. ; Sousa Passos, C.J. ; Sousa de Morais, S. ; Lebel, J. 2000. Methylmercury exposure affects motor performance of a riverine population of the Tapajos River, Brazilian Amazon. Int. Arch. Occup. Environ. Health, 73(3), 195–203.

Farella, N.; Lucote, M.; Louchouan, P.; Roulet, M. 2001. Deforestation modifying terrestrial organic transport in the Rio Tapajos, Brazilian Amazon. Organic Geochemestry, 32, 1443

Guimaraes, J.R.D.; Meili, M.; Hydlander, L.D.; Castro, E.S.; Roulet, M.; Mauro, J.B.N.; Lemos, R.A. 2000. Net mercury methylation in five tropical flood plain regions of Brazil: high in the rootzone of floating saprophytes mats but low in surface sediments and flooded soils. The Science of Total Environment, 261(1/3), 99–107

Guimaraes, J.R.D.; Roulet, M.; Lucotte, M.; Mergler, D. 2000. Mercury methylation along lake forest transect in the Tapajos River floodplain, Brazilian Amazon: seasonal and vertical variations. The Science of Total Environment, 261, 91–98

Lebel, J.; Mergler, D.; Branches, F.J.P.; Lucotte, M.; Amorim, M.; Larribe, F.; Dolbec, J. 1998. Neurotoxic effects of low level methylmercury contamination in the Amazon Basin. Environmental Research, 79(1), 20–32.

Lebel, J.; Mergler, D.; Lucotte, M.; Amorim, M.; Dolbec, J.; Miranda, D.; Arantès, G.; Rheault, I.; Pichet, P. 1996. Evidence of early nervous system dysfunction in Amazonian population exposed to lowlevels of methylmercury. Neurotoxicology, 17(1), 157–168.

Lebel, J.; Mergler, S.; Lucotte, M.; Dolbec, J. 1996. Mercury contamination. Ambio, 25(5), 374.

Lebel, J.; Roulet, M.; Mergler, D.; Lucotte, M.; Larribe, F. 1997. Fish diet and mercury exposure in a riparian amazonian population. Water, Air, and Soil Pollution, 97, 31–44.

Mergler, D. 2003. A tale of two rivers: a review of neurobehavioral deficits associated with consumption of fish from the Tapajos River (Para, Brazil) and the St. Lawrence River (Québec, Canada). Environmental Toxicology and Pharmacology, in press.

Mergler, D.; Bélanger, S.; Larribe, F.; Panisset, M.; Bowler, R.; Baldwin, M.; Lebel, J.; Hudnell, K. 1998. Preliminary evidence of neurotoxicity associated with eating fish from the Upper St. Lawrence River Lakes. NeuroToxicology 19, 691–702.

Roulet, M.; et al. 1998. The geochemistry of Hg in the Central Amazonian soils developed on the Alter-do-Chao formation of the lower Tapajos River valley, Para state Brazil. The Science of Total Environment, 223, 1–24.

Roulet, M.; Guimaraes, J.R.D.; Lucotte, M. 2001. Methylmecury production and accumulation in sediments and soils of an Amazonian floodplain effect of seasonal inundation. Water, Air and Soil Pollution, 128, 41–61.

Roulet, M.; Lucotte, M.; Canuel, R.; Farella, N.; Goch, Y.G.F.; Peleja, J.R.P.; Guimaraes, J.R.D.; Mergler, D.; Amorim, M. 2001. Spatio temporal geochemistry of Hg in waters of the Tapajos and

Amazon rivers, Brazil. Limnology and Oceanography, 46, 1158–1170.

Roulet, M.; Lucotte, M.; Canuel, R.; Farella, N.; Guimaraes, J.R.D.; Mergler, D.; Amorim, M. 2000. Increase in mercury contamination recorded in lacustrine sediments following deforestation in Central Amazonia. Chemical Geogology, 165, 243–266.

Roulet, M.; Lucotte, M.; Canuel, R.; Rheault, I.; Farella, N.; Serique, G.; Coelho, H.; Sousa Passos, C.J.; de Jesus da Silva, E.; Scavone de Andrade, P.; Mergler, D.; Guimaraes, J.R.D.; Amorim, M. 1998. Distribution and partition of total mercury in waters of the Tapajos River basin, Brazilian Amazonia. The Science of Total Environment, 213, 203–211.

Roulet, M.; Lucotte, M.; Farella, N.; Serique, G.; Coelho, H.; Sousa Passos, C.J.; de Jesus da Silva, E.; Scavone de Andrade, P.; Mergler, D.; Guimaraes, J.R.D.; Amorim, M. 1999. Effects of human colonization of the presence of mercury in the Amazonian ecosystems. Water, Air and Soil Pollution, 113, 297–313.

Roulet, J.; Lucotte, M.; Rheault, I.; Guimaraes, J.R.D. 2000. Methalylmercury in the water, seston and epiphyton of the Amazonian River and its flood plains, Tapajos River, Brazil. The Science of Total Environment, 261, 43–59.

Livestock and Agroecosystem Management for Community-based Integrated Malaria Control (East Africa)

Kabutha, C.; Mutero, C.; Kimani, V.; Gitau, G.; Kabuage, L.; Muthami, L.; Githure, J. 2002. Application of an ecosystem approach to human health in Mwea, Kenya: participatory methodologies for understanding local people's needs and perceptions. International Centre of Insect Physiology and Ecology, Nairobi, Kenya.

Mutero, C.M.; Kabutha, C.; Kimani, V.; Kabuage, L.; Gitau, G.; Ssennyonga, J.; Githure, J.; Muthami, L.; Kaida, A.; Musyoka, L.;

Kiarie, E.; Oganda, M. 2003. A transdisciplinary perspective of the links between malaria and agroecosystems in Kenya. International Centre of Insect Physiology and Ecology, Nairobi, Kenya.

Regional IDRC/Ford Ecosystem Approaches to Human Health Competition (Middle East and North Africa)

Kishk, F.M.; Gaber, H.M.; Abdallah, S.M. 2003. Environmental health risks reduction in rural Egypt: a holistic ecosystem approach. Paper presented at the 4th Annual Conference of the Global Development Network, 15–21 January 2003, Cairo, Egypt. **www.gdnet.org/pdf/Fourth_Annual_Conference/Parallels4/ GlobalizationHealthEnvironment/Kishk_paper.pdf**

Enhanced Human Well-being Through Livestock/Natural Resource Management (East African Highlands)

Jabbar, M.A.; Mohammed Saleem, M.A.; Li-Pun, H. 2001. Evolution towards transdisciplinarity in technology and resource management research: the case of a project in Ethiopia. In Klein, J.T.; Grossenbatcher-Mansuy, W.; Haberli, R.; Bail, A.; Scholz, R.; Myrtha Welti, A., ed., Transdisciplinarity: joint problem solving among science, technology and society. Birkhauser, Basel, Switzerland. pp. 172–167.

Jabbar, M.A.; Peden, D.; Mohamed Saleem, M.A.; Li-Pun, H., ed. 2000. Agroecosystems, natural resources management and human health related research in East Africa: proceedings of an international workshop held at ILRI, Addis Ababa, Ethiopia, 11–15 May 1998. ILRI, Addis Ababa, Ethiopia.

Jabbar, M.A.; Tekalign, M.; Mohamed Saleem, M.A. 2000. From plot to watershed management: experience in farmer participatory Vertisol technology generation and adoption in the Ethiopian Highlands. In Syers, J K.; Penning de Vries, F.W.T.; Nyamudeza, P., ed., The sustainable management of vertisols: IBSRAM Proceedings No. 20. CAB International, Wallingford, UK.

Okumu, B.; Jabbar, M.A.; Coleman, D.; Russel, N. 1999. Water conservation in the Ethiopian Highlands: application of a bioeconometric model. Paper presented at the open meeting of the Human Dimensions of Global Environmental Change Research Community, 24–26 June, Tokyo, Japan.

Okumu, B.; Jabbar, M.A.; Coleman, D.; Russel, N.; Mohammed Saleem, M.A.; Pender, J. 2000. Technology and policy impacts on economic performance, nutrients flows and soil erosion at the watershed level: the case of Ginchi in Ethiopia. Paper presented at the Global Development Network 2000 Conference, 11–14 December, Tokyo, Japan.

Urban Ecosystem Health (Nepal)

National Zoonoses and Food Hygiene Research Centre. 1999. Urban ecosystem health status in Ward 19–20 of Kathmandu. National Zoonoses & Food Hygiene Research Centre, Kathmandu, Nepal.

Technical publication of the National Zoonoses and Food Hygiene Research Centre and SAGUN, Kathmandu, Nepal:

➤ Tamang, B. 1999. Introduction to PAR–urban ecosystem health project and preliminary action plan.

➤ Tamang, B. 1999. Stakeholder's action plan and monitoring.

➤ REFLECT manual.

➤ Gender sensitization training manual.

➤ Urban ecosystem health awareness manual.

➤ Animal slaughtering and meat marketing practices in Nepal.

➤ Urban echinococosis in health transition in Nepal

Mapuche Environmental Resource Management

Duran Pérez, T. 2002. Antropologia interactiva: un estilo de antropologia aplicada en la IX Region de La Araucania, Chile. *In* CUHSO: cultura, hombre y sociedad. Centro de Estudios Socio-culturales, Universidad Catolica De Temuco, Temuco, Chile. pp. 23–57.

Duran Pérez, T.; Carrasco, N.; Prada, E. 2002. Acercamientos metodologicos hacia pueblos indigenas. Una exeriencia reflexionada desde La Araucania, Chile. Centro de Estudios Socio-culturales, Universidad Catolica de Temuco, Temuco, Chile.

Ecosystem Health (Tanzania)

Kilonzo, B.S.; Mvena, Z.S.K.; Machangu, R.S.; Mbise, T.J. 1997. Preliminary observations on factors responsible for long persistence and continued outbreaks of plague in Lushoto District, Tanzania. Acta Tropica, 68, 215–227.

Human Health and Changes in Potato Production Technology in the Highland Ecuadorian Agroecosystem

Anger, W.K.; Liang, Y.-X.; Nell, V.; Kang, S.-K.; Cole, D.C.; Bazylewicz-Walczak, B.; Rohlman, D.S.; Sizemore, O.J. 2000. Lessons learned: 15 years of the WHO-NCTB. Neurotoxicology, 21, 837–846.

Antle, J.; Stoorvogel, J.; Bowen, W.; Crissman, C.C.; Yanggen, D. 2003. Making an impact with impact assessment: the tradeoff analysis approach and lessons from the tradeoff project in Ecuador. Quarterly Journal of International Agriculture, in press.

Basantes, L. 1999. Reunion con grupo de mujeres, San Francisco de la Libertad. Sistematizacion, analisis e interpretacion de resultados. CIP-INIAP, San Gabriel, Ecuador.

Basantes, L.; Lopez, M.; Sherwood, S. 2000. Eco-Salud: case study on pesticide impacts in Carchi. Paper presented for the Andean Course on Ecologically Appropriate Agriculture, 9 October 2000, DSE/Germany.

Basantes, L.; Sherwood, S. 1999. Health and potato production in Carchi. Paper presented at the 2nd international meeting of the Global Initiative on Late Blight, 4–8 March 1999, Quito, Ecuador.

Berti, P.; Cole, D.C.; Crissman, C. 1999. Pesticides and health in potato production in highland Ecuador. Paper presented at the Ecosystem Approaches to Human Health Workshop, November 1999. CRDI/CSIH, Ottawa, ON, Canada.

CIP/INIAP. 1999. Impactos del uso de plaguicidas en al salud, produccion y medio ambiente en Carchi, Compendio de Investigaciones, Conferencia del 20 de octubre de 1999, Hostería Oasis, Ambuquí.

Cole, D.C.; Sherwood, S.; Crissman, C.C.; Barrera, V.; Espinosa, P. 2002. Pesticides and health in highland Ecuadorian potato production: assessing impacts and developing responses. International Journal of Occupational and Environmental Health, 8, 182–190.

Crissman, C.C. 1999. Impactos economicos del uso de plaguicidas en el cultivo de papa en la Provincia de Carchi. CIP-INIAP, Quito, Ecuador.

Crissman, C.C.; Yanggen, D.; Espinosa, P., ed. 2002. Los plaguicidas: impactos en production, salud, y medio embiente en Carchi, Ecuador. Abya Yala, Quito, Ecuador.

Espinosa, P. 1999. Estudio de línea base sobre el conocomiento y manejo de los pesticidas en el Carchi. CIP-INIAP, Quito, Ecuador.

McDermott, S.; Cole, D.C.; Krasevec, J.; Berti, P.; Ibrahim, S. 2002. Relationships between nutritional status and neurobehavioural function: implications for assessing pesticide effects among farming families in Ecuador. Poster presented at the First Annual Global Health Research Conference: Achieving Leadership in Global Health Research, 3–4 May 2002, Toronto, ON, Canada. University of Toronto, Toronto, ON, Canada.

Mera-Orcés, V. 2000. Agroecosystems management, social practices and health: a case study on pesticide use and gender in the Ecuadorian highlands. IDRC, Ottawa, ON, Canada.Technical report.

Mera-Orcés, V. 2001. Paying for survival with health: potato production practices, pesticide use and gender concerns in the Ecuadorian highlands. Journal of Agricultural Education and Extension, 8(1).

Paredes, M. 2001. We are like fingers of the same hand: a case study of peasant heterogeneity at the interface with technology and project intervention in Carchi, Ecuador. Wageningen University, Netherlands. MSc thesis.

Sherwood, S.; Basantes, L. 1999. Papas, pests, people, and power: addressing natural resource management conflict through policy interventions in Carchi, Ecuador. Paper presented at the conférence Ruralidad Sostenible Basada en la Participacion Ciudadana, 13–15 October 1999, Zamorano, Honduras.

Sherwood, S.; Larrea, S. 2001. Participatory methods: module for the MSc program in community-based natural resource management. Pontificate Catholic University of Ecuador.

Sherwood, S.; Nelson, R.; Thiele, G.; Ortiz, O. 2000. Farmer field schools in potato: a new platform for participatory training and research in the Andes, ILEA.

Thiele, G.; Nelson, R.; Ortiz, O.; Sherwood, S. 2001. Participatory research and training: ten lessons from farmer field schools in the Andes. Currents (Swedish University of Agricultural Sciences), 27, 4-11.

Viteri, H. 2000. Efectos neuropsicologicos del uso de plaguicidas en el Carchi. *In* INIAP et CIP, ed., Herramientoa de aprendizaje para facilitadores. INIAP/CIP, Quito, Ecuador.

Yanggen, D.; Crissman, C.C.; Espinosa, P., ed. 2002. Los plaguicidas: impactos en produccion, salud, y medio ambiente en Carchi. Abya Yala, Quito, Ecuador.

Environmental and Health Impacts of Small-scale Gold Mining in Ecuador

Funsad. 2001. A pequeña mineria del oro: impactos en el ambiente y la salud humana en la cuenca del puyango, sur del Ecuador. IDRC, Ottawa, ON, Canada. Final report (executive summary in English).

Manganese Exposure in General Population Resident in a Mining District, Mexico

Rodriguez, H.R.; Rios, C.; Rodriguez, Y.; Rosas, Y.; Siebe, C.; Ortiz, B. 2002. Impacto sobre la salud del ecosistema por las actividades antropogénicas en una cuenca manganesífera: avance de resultados, temporada de secas. ISAT.

Environmental and Social Performance Indicators and Sustainability Markers in Minerals Development

Echavarría Usher, C. 2003. Mining and indigenous peoples: contributions to an intellectual and ecosystem understanding of health and well-being. *In* Rapport, D.J.; Lasley, W.L.; Rolston, D.E.; Nielsen, N.O.; Qualset, C.O.; Damania, A.B., ed., Managing for healthy ecosystems. Lewis Publishers, Boca Raon, FL, USA. Chapter 86, pp. 863–880.

Maclean, C.; Warhurst, A.; Milner, P. 2003. Conceptual approaches to health and well-being minerals development: illustrations with the case of HIV/AIDS in southern Africa *In* Rapport, D.J.; Lasley, W.L.; Rolston, D.E.; Nielsen, N.O.; Qualset, C.O.; Damania, A.B., ed., Managing for healthy ecosystems. Lewis Publishers, Boca Raon, FL, USA. Chapter 85, pp. 843–862.

Mergler, D. 2003. Integrating human health into an ecosystem approach to mining. *In* Rapport, D.J.; Lasley, W.L.; Rolston, D.E.; Nielsen, N.O.; Qualset, C.O.; Damania, A.B., ed., Managing for healthy ecosystems. Lewis Publishers, Boca Raon, FL, USA. Chapter 87, pp. 881–890.

MERN (Mining and Energy Research Network). 2002. Environmental and social performance indicators (ESPIs) in minerals development. Final Report to the Department for International Development (DFID) and Mining and Energy Research Network (MERN) Club of Sponsors. University of Warwick, Warwick, UK.

Noronha, L. 2001. Designing tools to track health and well-being in mining regions of India. Natural Resources Forum, 25(1), 53–65.

Noronha, L. 2003. A conceptual framework for the development of tools to track health and well-being in a mining region: report from an Indian study. *In* Rapport, D.J.; Lasley, W.L.; Rolston, D.E.; Nielsen, N.O.; Qualset, C.O.; Damania, A.B., ed., Managing for healthy ecosystems. Lewis Publishers, Boca Raon, FL, USA. Chapter 88, pp. 891–904.

Urban Ecosystem and Human Health in Mexico City

Secretaría del Medio Ambiente. 2001. Ecosistema urbano y salud de los habitantes de la zona metropolitana del Valle de México. World Bank, Washington, DC, USA / Government of Mexico, Mexico DF, Mexico. **www.sma.df.gob.mx/publicaciones/aire/ ecosistema_urbano/ecosistema.htm**

Mexico Air Quality Management Team. 2002. Improving air quality in metropolitan Mexico City: an economic calculation. World Bank, Washington, DC, USA. Policy Research Working Paper 2785.

Rosales-Castillo, J.A.; Torres-Meza, V.M.; Olaiz-Fernández, G.; Borja-Aburto, V.H. 2001. Los efectos agudos de la contaminación del aire en la salud de la población evidencias de estudios epidemiológicos. Salud Publica Mexico, 43, 544–555. **www.insp.mx/salud/43/436_5.pdf**

Cicero-Fernandez, P.; Torres, V.; Rosales, A.; Cesar, H.; Dorland, K.; Muñoz, R.; Uribe, R.; Martinez, A.P. 2001. Evaluation of human exposure to ambient PM10 in the metropolitan area of Mexico City using a GIS-based methodology. Journal of the Air and Waste Management Association, 51, 1586–1593

Urban Ecosystem Health Indicators (Cuba)

Bonet, M.; Yassi, A.; Más, P.; Fernández, N.; Spiegel, J.M.; Concepción, M. 2001. Action research in Central Havana: the Cayo Hueso project. Paper presented at the 129th annual meeting of the American Public Health Association, 21–25 October 2001, Atlanta, GA, USA.

Fernandez, N.; Tate, R.; Bonet, M.; Canizares, M.; Más, P.; Yassi, A. 2000. Health-risk perception in the inner city community of Centro Habana, Cuba. International Journal of Occupational and Environmental Health, 6, 34–43.

Spiegel, J.M. 2002. Applying the ecosystem approach to human health. Paper presented at the International Population Health Conference, May 2002, Havana, Cuba.

Spiegel, J.M.; Beltran, M.; Chang, M.; Bonet, M. 2000. Measuring the costs and benefits of improvements to an urban ecosystem in a non-market setting: Conducting an economic evaluation of a community intervention in Centro Habana, Cuba. Paper presented at the conference of the International Society for Ecological Economics, 5–7 July 2000, Canberra, Australia.

Spiegel, J.M.; Bonet, M.; Yassi, A.; Más, P.; Tate, R. 2001. Social capital and health at a neighborhood level in Cuba. Paper presented at the 129th annual meeting of the American Public Health Association, 21–25 October 2001, Atlanta, GA, USA.

Spiegel, J.M.; Bonet, M.; Yassi, A.; Más, P.; Tate, R.; Fernandez, N. 2002. Action research to evaluate interventions in Central Havana. Paper presented at the 9th Canadian Conference on International Health, 27–30 October 2002, Ottawa, ON, Canada.

Spiegel, J.M.; Bonet, M.; Yassi, A.; Molina, E.; Concepción, M.; Más, P. 2001. Developing ecosystem health indicators in Centro Havana: a community-based approach. Ecosystem Health, 7(1), 15–26.

Spiegel, J.M.; Bonet, M.; Yassi, A.; Tate, R.; Concepción, M.; Más, P. 2001. Evaluating health interventions in Centro Habana. Paper presented at the 128th annual meeting of the American Public Health Association, 12–16 November, Boston, MA, USA.

Spiegel, J.M.; Yassi, A.; Bonet, M.; Concepcion, M.; Tate, R.B.; Canizares, M. 2003. Evaluating the effectiveness of interventions to improve health in the inner city community of Cayo Hueso. International Journal of Occupational and Environmental Health, in press.

Spiegel, J.M.; Yassi, A.; Tate, R. 2002. Dengue in Cuba: mobilisation against *Aedes aegypti*. The Lancet, Infections Diseases, 2, 204–205.

Tate, R.B.; Fernandez, N.; Canizares, M.; Bonet, M.; Yassi, A.; Más, P. 2000. Relationship between perception of community change and changes in health risk perception following community interventions in Central Havana. Paper presented at the

129th annual meeting of the American Public Health Association, 21–25 October 2001, Atlanta, GA, USA.

Tate, R.B.; Fernandez, N.; Yassi, A.; Canizares, M.; Spiegel, J.; Bonet, M. 2003. Changes in health risk perception following community intervention in Centro Habana. Health Promotion International, in press.

Yassi, A.; Fernandez, N.; Fernandez, A.; Bonet, M.; Tate, R.B.; Spiegel J. 2003. Community participation in a multi-sectoral intervention to address health determinants in an inner city community in Central Havana. Journal of Urban Health, in press.

Yassi, A.; Más, P.; Bonet, M.; Tate, R.B.; Fernández, N.; Spiegel, J.; Pérez, M. 1999. Applying an ecosystem approach to the determinants of health in Centro Havana. Ecosystem Health, 5(1), 3–19.

Recommendations and Future Directions

In the course of supporting research on the Ecohealth approach, IDRC has regulary worked with a number of partner orgaizations. More information can be found on their respective Web sites:

Canadian International Development Agency (CIDA): **www.acdi-cida.gc.ca**

Environment and Sustainable Development Unit, Faculty of Agriculture and Food Sciences, American University of Beirut: **staff.aub.edu.lb/~webeco/ESDU**

Instituto Nacional de Salud Publica (Mexico): **www.insp.mx**

John E. Fogarty International Centre for Advanced Study In the Health Sciences (USA): **www.fic.nih.gov**

National Institutes of Health (USA): **www.nih.gov**

Pan American Health Organization: **www.paho.org**

Special Programme for Research and Training in Tropical Diseases, World Health Organization: **www.who.int/tdr**

United Nations Environment Programme: **www.unep.org**

Université du Québec à Montréal (Canada): **www.uqam.ca**

University of Guelph (Canada): **www.uoguelph.ca**

World Bank: **www.worldbank.org**

World Health Organization: **www.who.int**

The Publisher

The International Development Research Centre is a public corporation created by the Parliament of Canada in 1970 to help researchers and communities in the developing world find solutions to their social, economic, and environmental problems. Support is directed toward developing an indigenous research capacity to sustain policies and technologies developing countries need to build healthier, more equitable, and more prosperous societies.

IDRC Books publishes research results and scholarly studies on global and regional issues related to sustainable and equitable development. As a specialist in development literature, IDRC Books contributes to the body of knowledge on these issues to further the cause of global understanding and equity. The full catalogue is available at **www.idrc.ca/booktique**.